Third Edition

Handbook of
Health Assessment

Ellen B. Rudy, RN, PhD, FAAN
Professor and Dean
School of Nursing
University of Pittsburgh
Pittsburgh, Pennsylvania

V. Ruth Gray, EdD, RN
Professor and Associate Dean, Graduate Program
University of Akron
College of Nursing
Akron, Ohio

APPLETON & LANGE
Norwalk, Connecticut

0-8385-3602-6

Notice: Our knowledge in clinical sciences is constantly changing. As new information becomes available, changes in treatment and in the use of drugs become necessary. The authors and the publisher of this volume have taken care to make certain that the doses of drugs and schedules of treatment are correct and compatible with the standards generally accepted at the time of publication. The reader is advised to consult carefully the instruction and information material included in the package insert of each drug or therapeutic agent before administration. This advice is especially important when using new or infrequently used drugs.

Prentice Hall International (UK) Limited, *London*
Prentice Hall of Australia Pty. Limited, *Sydney*
Prentice Hall Canada, Inc., *Toronto*
Prentice Hall Hispanoamericana, S.A., *Mexico*
Prentice Hall of India Private Limited, *New Delhi*
Prentice Hall of Japan, Inc., *Tokyo*
Simon & Schuster Asia Pte. Ltd., *Singapore*
Editora Prentice Hall do Brasil Ltda., *Rio de Janeiro*
Prentice Hall, *Englewood Cliffs, New Jersey*

Library of Congress Cataloging-in-Publication Data
Rudy, Ellen B.
  Handbook of health assessment / Ellen B. Rudy, V. Ruth
Gray. -- 3rd ed.
    p.   cm.
  Includes index.
  ISBN 0-8385-3602-6
  1. Nursing diagnosis.   I. Gray, V. Ruth.   II. Title.
RT48.6.R83   1991   91-12044
616.07′54   -dc20   CIP

Acquisitions Editor: William Brottmiller
Production Editor: Elizabeth Ryan
Designer: Michael Kelly

PRINTED IN THE UNITED STATES OF AMERICA

Contents

Preface

The third edition of this book comes at a time when nursing diagnoses are being viewed from a classification schema (taxonomy) that represents a unitary person framework. The richness and clearly more wholistic perspective this brings to the traditional history and physical format provides practitioners with data that they can easily use to collaborate with physician colleagues, and data that can be used to make independent nursing diagnoses and decisions.

We have tried to keep this book small but detailed enough to give you the guidance you need in the clinical setting. Again, we urge you to *use* the book—write in it, underline it, add new material or information as you find it. The sections on infants and children, adolescents, and the elderly have purposely been kept concise and present only the health history and physical examination as they differ from the adult.

Our sincere thanks go to our colleagues who have used our book and have provided excellent suggestions to Appleton & Lange for judging it worthy of another edition.

We acknowledge the help of our families, colleagues and students, each of whom have contributed to making this book a reality.

Ellen B. Rudy, PhD, RN, FAAN
V. Ruth Gray, EdD, RN

Introduction

This book is designed to guide the reader in attaining proficiency in the content and skills necessary to do health assessments on patients and clients. The purpose of a health assessment includes an evaluation of present health status including screening for specific disease conditions, assessment of a constellation of signs and symptoms that identify a pathological condition, monitoring of the progress of treatment and care, and determining physiological and psychological levels of health. As nurses have incorporated health assessment skills into their practice they have not only broadened their own data base for planning care, but have helped to focus on the wholistic view of the patient. Nursing then seeks to promote and maintain health, work collaboratively with the physician in the diagnosis and treatment of disease, and provide independent nursing care based on nursing diagnosis.

By making such a statement, it is clear that we (the authors) view nursing as having both interdependent and independent functions. Historically nurses have spent a considerable portion of their time in interdependent responsibilities exercising clinical judgment in the *execution* of established medical protocols. More recently nurses have focused on independent responsibilities exercising clinical judgment in the *formulation* and *use* of nursing diagnosis. The expansion of assessment skills enables the nurse to be even more effective in interdependent and independent functioning.

Both types of functioning are particularly evident in

clinical settings where nurses are responsible for an initial health history and physical examinations and physicians are responsible for medical diagnosis and treatment. For this reason the health history format in this book has been expanded to include patient information that can be used for making both medical and nursing diagnoses.

In the past two decades the conceptualization and use of nursing diagnosis have undergone major changes. With leadership from the North American Nursing Diagnosis Association (NANDA) the number of nursing diagnoses has increased, the use of nursing diagnoses has spread, and the development of a classification scheme (taxonomy) has evolved. It is clear that continual change will occur within the nursing diagnoses movement in nursing, and it is beyond the scope of this book to provide a complete discussion and description of nursing diagnoses. However, because a health assessment assumes that the nurse will make a clinical judgment about a patient, based on subjective and objective data, the most recent organization and proposed taxonomy for nursing diagnoses are listed below. A nursing diagnosis, like a medical diagnosis, cannot be made until a constellation of specific signs and symptoms is present. As always, intuition can play a role in deciding when to look for symptoms (e.g., what lab studies to order or what questions to ask), but intuition alone without supporting data is little more than guessing.

The present classification system used by NANDA is based on nine identified Human Response Patterns representing unitary man. These nine patterns are Choosing, Communicating, Exchanging, Feeling, Knowing, Moving, Perceiving, Relating and Valuing.

The definitions of these Human Response Patterns are as follows:

Choosing. To select between alternates; the action of selecting or exercising preference in regard to a matter in which one is a free agent; to determine in favor of a course; to decide in accordance with inclinations.

Communicating. To converse; to impart, confer, or transmit thoughts, feelings, or information, internally or externally, verbally or nonverbally.

Exchanging. To give, relinquish, or lose something while receiving something in return; the substitution of one element for another; the reciprocal act of giving and receiving.

Feeling. To experience a consciousness, sensation, apprehension, or sense; to be consciously or emotionally affected by a fact, event, or state.

Knowing. To recognize or acknowledge a thing or a person; to be familiar with by experience or through information or report; to be cognizant of something through observation, inquiry, or information; to be conversant with a body of facts, principles, or methods of action; to understand.

Moving. To change the place or position of a body or any member of the body; to put and/or keep in motion; to provoke an excretion or discharge; the urge to action or to do something; to take action.

Perceiving. To apprehend with the mind; to become aware of by the senses; to apprehend what is not open or present to observation; to take in fully or adequately.

Relating. To connect, to establish a link between, to stand in some association to another thing, person, or place; to be borne or thrust in between things.

Valuing. To be concerned about, to care; the worth or worthiness; the relative status of a thing, or the estimate in which it is held, according to its real or supposed worth, usefulness, or importance; one's opinion of liking for a person or thing; to equate in importance.

The specific nursing diagnoses are all organized into the classification scheme (taxonomy) of these nine patterns and are listed below. These diagnoses are considered conditions that necessitate nursing care and are patient responses which nurses can independently treat.

TAXONOMY OF NURSING DIAGNOSIS BY HUMAN RESPONSE PATTERNS*

I.   *Human Response Pattern: Choosing*
    A. Family Coping, Impaired
       1. Compromised
       2. Disabled
    B. [Health Seeking Behavior]
       1. Health Seeking Behaviors, (Specify)
    C. Individual Coping, Impaired
       1. Adjustment, Impaired
       2. Conflict: Decisional
       3. Coping: Defensive
       4. Denial, Impaired
       5. Noncompliance

II. *Human Response Pattern: Communicating*
    A. [Communication, Impaired]
       1. Verbal

III. *Human Response Pattern: Exchanging*
    A. [Bowel Elimination, Altered]
       1. Bowel Incontinence
       2. Constipation: Colonic
       3. Constipation: Perceived
       4. Diarrhea

NOTES: Items in brackets are not NANDA accepted diagnoses.
Items with an asterisk (*) are changes in terminology from NANDA diagnostic labels.
NANDA diagnoses not specifically identified are embedded in the coding system.
Sources: Fitzpatrick et al., 1989 and the North American Nursing Diagnosis Association (NANDA), 1989.

B. Cardiac Output, Altered
C. [Fluid Volume, Altered]
    1. Deficit
    2. Deficit: Risk
    3. Excess
D. Injury: Risk
    1. Aspiration
    2. Disuse Syndrome
    3. Poisoning
    4. Suffocation
    5. Trauma
E. [Nutrition, Altered]
    1. Less than Body Requirement
    2. More than Body Requirement
    3. More than Body Requirement: Risk
F. [Physical Regulation, Altered]
    1. Dysreflexia
    2. Hyperthermia
    3. Hypothermia
    4. Infection: Risk
    5. Thermoregulation, Impaired
G. [Respiration, Altered]
    1. Airway Clearance, Impaired
    2. Breathing Pattern, Impaired
    3. Gas Exchange, Impaired
    4. Protection, Altered
H. Tissue Integrity, Altered
    1. Oral Mucous Membranes, Impaired
    2. Skin Integrity, Impaired
    3. Skin Integrity, Impaired: Risk
I. [Tissue Perfusion, Altered]
    1. Cardiopulmonary
    2. Cerebral
    3. Gastrointestinal
    4. Peripheral
    5. Renal

IX.   *Human Response Pattern: Valuing*
    A.   [Spiritual State, Altered]
        1.   Spiritual Distress

Two new nursing diagnoses have not been placed in the taxonomic structure but may be used as diagnosis. They are: Effective breastfeeding, Altered protection.

In each chapter of the physical assessment a normal and abnormal write-up is provided. In most cases additional data are needed to formulate nursing diagnoses. The etiology for each nursing diagnosis is determined by the findings from the patient's individual situation. Each diagnosis is based on the identification of the appropriate defining characteristics. In order to assist the nurse to incorporate nursing diagnoses in the total assessment we have provided those nursing diagnoses that would commonly occur with these abnormal findings.

The taking of a medical history and performing a physical examination have been the hallmark of medical diagnosis since the beginning of medical education. In order to provide consistency between medical practitioners, the elements of the history and physical examination have become standardized. For example, the Medical History always starts with the Chief Complaint, followed by the History of the Present Illness and so forth. As more and more nurses have been introduced to this routine of a health history and physical examination they have incorporated these skills into their patient assessments.

With the increasing interest in nursing diagnosis as a means of explicating those responses which nurses can independently treat, there is a trend away from what is considered the "medical model" of a history and physical assessment to new formats for patient assessment. It is appropriate for nurses functioning in a specialized area of nursing to develop their own assessment tools aimed at determining appropriate nursing diagnoses.

The purpose of this book, however, is to teach the standard history and physical format used by medicine so that a consistent data base on patients can be obtained that is useful to both nurses and physicians. In order to broaden the data base for determining appropriate nursing diagnoses for each patient, the Health History has been expanded under the heading, Patient Profile. Nurses using this format find they can provide assessment data useful to physicians as well as formulate nursing diagnoses for their patients.

1 | Outline of Health History

Before beginning the actual health history, identifying information should be obtained from the patient or other reliable source. This includes the following:

Name
Address
Phone Number
Social Security Number
Sex
Birth Date
Marital Status
Occupation
Next of Kin

The interviewing skills of the examiner will determine to a large degree how complete and accurate the health history data base will be. The first step in effective communication is establishing a rather quick rapport with the patient that conveys a caring, listening attitude. When eliciting a health history keep the following points in mind.

Privacy for the Interview

This may be limited to pulling the curtain around the patient's cubicle or asking visitors to step outside. Whatever gesture is necessary, patients are more likely to give accurate, instead of socially acceptable, answers when they feel others cannot hear them.

Show Interest in the Patient

The point to be made here is that using direct eye contact, keeping track of what the patient has already said, and allowing the patient adequate time to "tell his story," all imply interest by the examiner and will usually produce a more cooperative atmosphere.

Validate Conclusions

As the patient describes symptoms or specific health problems, the examiner may want to validate what she has been hearing to make sure the patient agrees with the examiner's conclusion or understanding of the situation.

Be Aware of Missing or Conflicting Information

The information necessary to make a diagnosis or validate a health problem is not always forthcoming in the health history. The examiner will often need to ask the same questions in a variety of ways to get any clear understanding of what is happening to the patient. In fact, new practitioners will occasionally find that the practiced examiner can elicit new information from the patient just by altering the wording of a question.

Avoid Medical Terminology

Medical jargon and terminology, while readily understood by other health care professionals, is not appropriate for communicating with a patient. Lay terms should be used when asking questions and at times "street language" will be necessary to communicate adequately with the patient.

Listen Without Bias or Judgment

A health history will reveal many things about a person's life style, behaviors, and attitudes. Even when the patient reveals aspects of his or her life that you find repulsive or distressing, any judgments you convey to the patient may interfere with future communication or rapport. The purpose of the health history is to get a data base for making judgments on health or illness. This is more easily done in a nonjudgmental atmosphere.

Be Professional in Appearance and Behavior

The examiner must be constantly aware that appearance, manner of asking questions, and nonverbal forms of communication all contribute to the way the patient views the examiner. A professional presentation gives patients confidence in the care that they will receive and often contributes to more open communication.

Protect Yourself and Your Patient From Transmittable Diseases

It goes without saying, whenever you are required to examine a patient you will be in intimate contact with the person's skin, mucous membranes, and possible body secretions. Hand washing before beginning the physical examination is standard procedure. Additional hand washing is done following examination of lymph nodes of axilla and following examination of the genital area. Anytime that you are exposed to body secretions (such as in the rectal and genital exams), ulcerations, wounds, or areas with drainage, examiners should protect themselves and their clothing. This means wearing latex gloves and in some cases a cover gown that can be removed and washed.

The widespread acceptance of Body Substance Isolation as a precaution against the spread of acquired immunocompromised disease syndrome (AIDS) should be the guiding principle to prevent the spread of all communicable diseases.

I. CHIEF COMPLAINT AND ITS DURATION (CC)

This, in brief, is the answer in the patient's own words to the question "What brought you here today?" The chief complaint should be in one sentence, and include the duration of the problem or symptom if possible. The reason for the visit may also be a routine physical or well checkup.

Reliability

At this point a note should be made as to whether the history was obtained from the patient, relative, friend or physician, the mental condition of the patient, and the probable reliability of the history.

II. HISTORY OF PRESENT ILLNESS (HPI)

This is a well-organized, chronological elaboration of the patient's chief complaint from the time of onset until he or she is seen by you. Describe as accurately as possible the course of the present illness. This history includes:

>   Duration of symptom or problem
>   Onset:
>   Date
>   Manner (e.g., sudden, gradual)
>   Precipitating or predisposing factors
>   Characteristics and course of symptom or problem
>   Location (anatomical)
>   Quality
>   Quantity
>   Timing (what time of day does it occur?)
>   Setting
>   Factors that alleviate, including medication (what makes it better?); factors that aggravate (what makes symptom worse?)
>   Associated factors

Ask the patient, "When were you last your normal self?"

The course of the disease should be developed symptomatically in chronological order, each symptom thoroughly developed in its course. When there is a conspicuous disturbance of a particular organ or system, questions should be asked about possible symptoms that refer to the disturbance of this organ or system. A particular pattern of symptoms may suggest a particular disease state. When this occurs it becomes important to ask specific questions about commonly associated symptoms so that a diagnosis is more easily established.

For example, if a patient comes to you for increased shortness of breath during routine activities, you should establish the description of this symptom, its progress, etc., according to the HPI format. This should be followed by specific questions related to the respiratory and cardiovascular systems to more clearly delineate the possible cause of the symptom.

More detailed history questions related to each body system are presented at the beginning of each chapter in the physical examination portion of the book.

Inquiry should be made concerning any general abnormality and symptoms beyond those already mentioned, e.g., pain, chills, fever, night sweats, weight loss, anorexia, tremors.

Included, finally, is a statement of any continuing problem, i.e., diabetes, obesity, hypertension, heart disease.

III. PAST HISTORY (PH)

General Health
Statement of health prior to examination.

Medical History
Previous major illnesses. Diagnoses. Dates. Hospitalization. Complications. Physician.

Surgical History
Procedures. Dates. Complications. Hospitals and physicians.

Other Hospitalizations
Diagnoses. Dates. Treatments. Physicians. The purpose of this question is to elicit information not covered through medical and surgical past history. Specific reference should be made to any past traumas or accidents and any past psychiatric illnesses.

Injuries and Resulting Disabilities

Allergy
Asthma, hay fever, hives, poison oak, food idiosyncracy, drugs and reactions. Previous penicillin treatment.

Acute Infectious Diseases
Acute streptococcal infections, rheumatic fever, mononucleosis, hepatitis.

If other infections should be mentioned, specific statements must be made concerning them; if there is a history of any acute infections, the duration, severity, complications, and sequelae should be recorded. Inquire about childhood diseases and immunizations for polio, measles, mumps, whooping cough, chicken pox, diphtheria, tetanus. Also inquire about unusual reactions to immunizations.

Medications
Currently taken and past reactions. Include both prescription and over-the-counter drugs.

Drugs
Do you presently have a drug habit? Which drug: cocaine, marijuana, heroin, "speed," alcohol, etc.? Have you ever tried to stop taking drugs? Have you ever shared a needle with another person?

IV. FAMILY HISTORY (FH)

A family-tree diagram is helpful in recording this information. This diagram will indicate the present health of each family member, note age, sex, and whether alive or deceased—and mark the incidence of hereditary diseases. The family tree may include grandparents if familial diseases are identified. Specific inquiry should be made about hereditary and communicable diseases such as diabetes, cystic fibrosis, hemophilia, heart disease, hypertension, obesity, cancer, and tuberculosis. Suggested family-tree symbols:

♀ = female   ♂ = male   X = deceased

Example: Patient is a 35-year-old male with diabetes mellitus. His mother is 67 years old, living and well; his father died at age 52 from heart disease; two sisters, ages 34 and 36, are living and well.

```
♀ _____ ♂
67                                  52
      ♂        ♀        ♀          heart disease
      35       34       36
      pt DM    L&W      L&W
```

V. REVIEW OF SYSTEMS (ROS)

This part of the history reviews major symptoms as they relate to general body systems. Symptoms revealed may "paint a picture" for clues relating to the patient's present illness. Remember these are *patient* responses and *not physical findings.*

Recall that more detailed history questions for each body system are at the beginning of each chapter in the physical examination sections.

Skin
Rash, eruptions, itching, pigmentation change, texture change, moisture, hair growth.

Nails
Color changes, brittleness, curvature.

Head and Scalp
Headaches, dizziness, syncope, vertigo; hair color, texture, and distribution; scalp itching or lesions.

Eyes
Vision, color blindness, diplopia, trauma, inflammatory disease, pain, recent refraction (last exam), need for glasses, contact lenses.

Ears
Hearing, earache, discharge, tinnitus, vertigo.

Nose and Sinuses
Sense of smell, colds, obstruction, epistaxis, postnasal drip, sinus pain.

Mouth and Teeth
Lesions, soreness, pain, bleeding or receding gums, abscesses, teeth extractions, chewing surfaces, dentures, difficulty chewing or swallowing, last dental exam.

Throat and Neck
Sore throats, tonsillitis, hoarseness, neck swelling, stiffness, or pain.

Breasts
Pain, tenderness, lumps, discharge, changes, breast feeding, gynecomastia. Do you know how to do self-breast examination (SBE)? How often do you do it?

Respiratory
Pain in chest, dyspnea at rest or with exercise, wheezing cough, sputum (character and quantity), hemoptysis, night sweats, orthopnea, paroxysmal nocturnal dyspnea, last x-ray of chest and result, including where obtained.

Cardiovascular
Pain or distress over precordium, radiation of pain, palpitation, changes in rate of rhythm, dyspnea, orthopnea, edema, cyanosis, estimate of exercise tolerance, blood pressure, if known, claudication, varicose veins, phlebitis, last EKG and result, including where obtained.

Gastrointestinal
Appetite and digestion, change in weight, pain with relation to swallowing or eating, eructation, flatulence, heartburn, nausea, vomiting, hematemesis, usual bowel elimination pattern, cathartics, diarrhea, stools (clay colored, tarry, fresh blood), hemorrhoids, hernia, jaundice, dark urine, use of antacids.

Genitourinary
Usual urinary elimination pattern, color, dysuria, pain, passage of gravel, frequency, nocturia, hematuria, polydipsia, polyuria, oliguria, edema of face, hesitance, dribbling, loss in size and force of stream.

Sexuality
Sexual preference, number of sexual partners. Sexual adjustment, satisfaction with life style. History of gonorrhea, syphilis or herpes. Inquire by name (many use street language, e.g., clap). Symptoms, treatment (self or medical), re-infection, present status. Diagnosis of HIV infection (AIDS) or chronic lymphadenopathy syndrome (AIDS-related complex). Sexual relationship with anyone diagnosed with AIDS or AIDS-related complex (ARC).

Males
Onset of puberty, voice change, erections, emissions, satisfactory sexual adjustment, any effect of illness on sexuality. Do you practice self-exam of testicles? How often?

Females
Age of menarche, cycle description, dysmenorrhea (primary or secondary), last menstrual period, climacteric symptoms, douching practices, last Pap test, vaginal discharge, medications. Pregnancies (number, problems, complications) infertility problems, type of contraception, dyspareunia, satisfactory sexual adjustment, any effect of illness on sexuality.

Musculoskeletal
Morning stiffness, backache, pain, joint swelling, muscular

weakness or atrophy, cramps, limitation of movement.

Neurological
Nervousness, insomnia, drowsiness, vertigo, tremors, convulsions, paralysis, paresthesia, neuralgia, memory, orientation, affect.

Lymphatic
Swollen lymph nodes, pain. Chronic, systemic swollen or tender lymph nodes.

Hematopoietic
Anemia, tendency to bruise or bleed, thrombosis, thrombophlebitis, blood transfusions and reactions.

Endocrine
Relative size of body including back, feet and head, hair distribution and texture, enlargement of thyroid, intolerance to heat or cold, weakness, exophthalmia, tremor, polyphagia, polydipsia, polyuria, glycosuria.

Ask the patient these general questions at the end of the history"

"Is there anything else that concerns you?"
"What problem concerns you the most?"

VI. PATIENT PROFILE

These questions are intended to address some of the subjective data needed to assess the nursing diagnoses from the nine human response patterns. Additional data will be obtained from other parts of the health history and the physical examination (PE). The format for this part of the history is based in part on the prototype provided by Guzzetta, Bunter, Prinkey, Sherer, and Seifert (1989). Suggested questions are listed for each response pattern; statements in parentheses are to be answered by the examiner. Objective data to be obtained from the physical exam are marked as **PE**.

Human Response Patterns	**Nursing Diagnoses (potential or altered)**

Communicating. A pattern involving sending messages
Can you read and write English? Any other languages?
(Are speech problems evident; are alternate forms for communication used?)
	Communication
	  Verbal
	  Nonverbal

Valuing. A pattern involving the assigning of relative worth
Religion and its importance in your life (will illness interfere with religious practices?) Ethnic background? (explore cultural beliefs concerning health practices and illness)
	Spiritual State
	  Distress
	  Despair

Relating. A pattern involving establishing bonds
Role
  Marital status?
  Health of spouse or significant other?
  (Number of children)
  Importance of family, support?
  Occupation, importance of work?
  Financial situation?
  Impact of illness on family/finances?
	Role Performance
	  Parenting
	  Sexual dysfunction
	  Work
	  Family
	  Social/leisure
	  Family processes

Sexual relations (satisfactory/unsatisfactory) Risk preference group for AIDS? bisexual, homosexual, multiple partners	Sexual Patterns

Impact of illness on sexual relations?

Socialization

Importance of close friends?   Impaired Social
Usual social and leisure activities   Interaction
                                       Social isolation
                                       Social withdrawal

Knowing. A pattern involving the
meaning associated with information

(Does the patient understand his   Knowledge Deficit
or her present health state? Does
the patient have any unrealistic
expectations of therapy? Any
misconceptions?)

What important things do you do
to keep healthy?

Exposure to toxins, pollution?

Foreign travel and military service?

Any use of alcohol, tobacco, drugs?

Educational level

What is your best way to learn;   Learning Problems
any difficulty learning?

(This will be evaluated in neuro   Thought Processes
PE and includes level of alert-
ness, orientation, memory, and
appropriateness of behaviors
and responses to questions)

Feeling. A pattern involving the
subjective awareness of information,
both physical and emotional.

Physical Comfort

(Information on pain and com-   Comfort
fort will be primarily evaluated   Pain/chronic
in Chief Complaint and History   Pain/acute
of Present Illness)   Discomfort

Emotional Comfort

What activities, events or people   Anxiety
in your life produce tension?   Fear

Have you had a recent stressful life event?

How do you usually handle big problems?

Anticipatory grieving
Dysfunctional grieving
Posttrauma response
Rape trauma syndrome
Rape trauma syndrome: Compound reaction
Rape trauma syndrome: Silent reaction
Risk of violence

Moving. A pattern involving activity

Activity

(Physical disability, limitations of movement, weaknesses will be evaluated in ROS and PE of musculoskeletal system

Describe routine activity/exercise (type, pattern, regularity) including exercise in leisure time.

Impaired physical ability
Altered growth and development

Do you have sufficient energy for necessary/desired activity?

Activity intolerance

Describe any impairments or limitations you have.

Self-care deficits

Can you function independently or with help? How much help?

Bathing
Dressing
Grooming
Feeding

Sleep/Rest

Describe sleep patterns (time to bed, hours of sleep, difficulty getting or staying asleep, time of awakening, feeling rested after sleep):

Sleep pattern disturbance

Any aids to induce sleep?

Recreation

Describe usual leisure and social activities.

Deficit in diversional activity

Home Maintenance

What size home (apartment, etc.) do you live in? Does it have a bathroom? stairs?

Altered home maintenance

What are your responsibilities at home?

Impaired home maintenance management

Health Maintenance

How do you view your present health?

Altered health management

What important things do you do to keep healthy?

Any difficulty following nurse/ physician suggestions or therapeutic regimen?

Perceiving. A pattern involving the reception of information

Describe yourself and how you feel about yourself:

Altered self-concept
Body image disturbance

Has your illness caused any changes in how you feel about yourself or your body?

Personal identity disturbance
Self-esteem disturbance:
  Chronic low
  Situational
Hopelessness
Powerlessness

(Will be assessed in PE)

Altered sensory/ perception
  Visual
  Auditory
  Kinesthetic
  Gustatory

Tactile
Olfactory

Exchanging. A pattern involving mutual giving and receiving (Except for nutrition and elimination, this pattern will be assessed during the PE. Questions on elimination are addressed with the Review of Symptoms.)

Typical daily food intake
Typical daily fluid intake
Dietary supplements
Weight loss/gain (amount, time span)
Any appetite changes?

Alteration in nutrition
More than body requirements

Less than body requirements

Any food allergies?
Caffeine intake

VII. RECORDING

The following is an example of a health history.

Name:	Ruth Wanone
Address:	7712 Straight Lane
	Newton Falls, Michigan
Telephone:	489-1785
Social Security Number:	285-37-7920
Sex:	Female
Birthdate:	4/13/24 Age: 67
Marital Status:	Widow
Occupation:	Homemaker
Height:	4'10-1/2"
Weight:	156 lbs.
Next of Kin:	Mother (83 years old)
Address:	Same
Date:	September 8, 1991

Chief Complaint (CC):

"Bad pain in my chest for 1-1/2 hours yesterday."

History of Present Illness (HPI)

This 67-year-old white, widowed female had an episode of stabbing midsternal chest pain, 1 day ago (9/7/91). While she was reading, the pain radiated to the left arm and jaw and was accompanied by a feeling of tightness and pressure in the chest. No diaphoresis, nausea, vomiting, dizziness or shortness of breath. Pain unrelieved with positioning, took Isordil 10mg × 2, 20 min apart. Pain finally relieved 1½ hours later. Second onset of pain occurred early today while patient was sitting down to eat breakfast. Pain was same character as the day before, no accompanying symptoms. Isordil 10mg taken every 30 min × 3; pain relieved after 2 hours. Went to physician's office after pain stopped and ECG showed an acute myocardial infarction. Admitted to coronary care unit from physician's office. Has been diagnosed with coronary artery disease with angina since 1971. Takes Isordil 10mg qid and hs. Diabetes mellitus since 1968, treated with Diabinese 100mg in am, 150mg in pm. No history of hypertension.

Past History (PH)

Childhood Illnesses	Had measles, mumps, chicken pox; no history of rheumatic fever.
Immunizations	Usual childhood immunizations, does not remember specifics.
Medical History	Psoriasis since 1975
	Diabetes mellitus since 1968
	Coronary artery disease and heart murmur 1975
	Osteoarthritis of knees and hips 1978
Surgical History	Umbilical herniorrhaphy and appendectomy in 1962 Dr. Bix, East Suburban Hospital, Michigan

	Heart cath. 1975 Dr. Horn, East Suburban Hospital
	Coronary artery bypass graft (single graft) 1975, Dr. Horn, East Suburban Hospital
	Total hip replacement L hip 1976 Dr. John Cleary, East Suburban Hospital
Traumas/Injuries	Only minor ones
Allergies	None
Medications	Diabenese 100mg am, 150mg, pm (afternoon)
	Motrin 400mg qid pc
	Isordil 10mg qid & hs
	Valisone ointment prn for psoriasis
	Ionill shampoo prn for psoriasis
	Milk of Magnesia 2 T prn for constipation

Family History
Strong family history of CAD. Does not know grandparents' history.

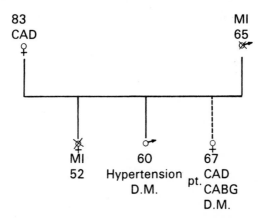

Review of Systems (ROS)

Skin
Has periodic flareups of psoriasis with patchy, red, scaly areas scattered on back, calves, and scalp. Presently has areas on front of scalp and back. Treats with OTCD for skin and shampoo for scalp.

Nails
No problems with brittleness; no color changes.

Head and Scalp
Denies headaches, dizziness or syncope. Hair somewhat thinner in recent years, no scalp lesions.

Eyes
Does not wear corrective glasses, last exam 1982, no pain, tearing, itching, no visual problems.

Ears
No difficulty hearing, no discharge, tinnitus or lesions.

Nose and Sinuses
Infrequent colds, no sinus problems, no epistaxis.

Mouth and Teeth
No dentures, cavities filled, no bleeding gums, no problems chewing or swallowing. Last dental exam 6 months ago.

Throat and Neck
Raw sore throat, no problems with hoarseness, stiffness, pain or neck swelling.

Breasts
No lumps, discharge, or pain. Does self-breast exam on an irregular basis.

Respiratory
No coughing, wheezing or hemoptysis. Sleeps on 1 pillow, last chest x-ray 1990, some dyspnea ⁻ith stair climbing for past 4 years. Exercise limited more by arthritis than by respirations.

Cardiovascular and Peripheral Vascular
Has occasional midsternal pain with exertion (see HPI for recent occurrence). Takes Isordil 10mg with chest pain. Had prescription for sublingual nitroglycerine but did not have prescription filled. No palpitations, orthopnea, cyanosis. No edema of feet or hands. No paroxysmal nocturnal dyspnea.

Gastrointestinal
No problems with eating, no heartburn, diarrhea, nausea or vomiting. Uses laxative (Milk of Magnesia) occasionally (once a month) for constipation.

Genitourinary
No pain or burning with voiding. Urine clear yellow. Voids about 6× a day and 2× at night. Gravida ii Para ii. Last menstrual period at 49, no problem with menopause. Last Pap test 1989 (normal). No vaginal discharge or itching. Is not sexually active since death of husband. No history of sexually transmitted diseases. Not a member of high risk group for HIV infection.

Musculoskeletal
Stiffness in back of left leg upon awakening. Fingers and knees are painful with some swelling in winter months. No muscle weakness.

Neurological
No numbness or tingling in extremities, no tremors, convulsions, loss of memory or loss of consciousness. No history of mental illness. Admits to excessive nervousness at times in stressful situations.

Lymphatic
No swollen or painful nodes.

Hematopoietic
No bruising or thrombophlebitis. Had multiple blood transfusions with CABG surgery, no reactions.

Endocrine
Known diabetic but denies any symptoms of polydipsia, polyphasia, or polyuria. Does not do urine testing at home. Goes to MD every 3 months for blood work. No enlargement of thyroid, no intolerance to heat or cold.

Patient Profile

Communicating
No problem with communication.

Valuing
Patient is Catholic but does not attend church regularly and does not feel that religion is very important in her life. She is of Italian descent many generations ago.

Relating
Has been a widow for 18 years, has two daughters who live in town but not in same neighborhood. Patient's 83-year-old mother lives with the patient, and at present the mother is in good health and able to manage her own care. Patient is head of her own household but relies heavily on her children and their families for handling problems and for emotional support. She has several close friends from the Golden Agers' Club and the Homemakers' Club who call several times a week.

Knowing
Appears to understand her present health status. Is frightened she might die suddenly and leave her mother with no one to

care for her. Is a high school graduate; learns new material best by demonstration. Watches TV several hours a day, reads newspapers and occasionally magazines.

Feeling

In no acute pain at present; generally when she encounters pain she tries to ignore it, does not take any medication for pain and usually does not tell anyone about it.

Tension-producing situations include family illness and entertaining company at her home. She becomes nervous when getting the house and food ready for company. Her children are the biggest help in dealing with stress. She tries to avoid stressful situations when possible or else removes herself from whatever is causing the stress. Recent major life change was breast malignancy of her 46-year-old daughter. Daughter has recovered from mastectomy and has not required chemotherapy or radiation.

The present hospital admission for a heart attack is very upsetting because of her fear for herself and her mother.

Moving

Does primarily sedentary activities including TV watching, crocheting, playing cards, and reading. Occasionally does some gardening. Considers housework as sufficient exercise; does consider arthritis in her knees as an inhibitor of more exercise. Has sufficient energy for desired activities but does take daily afternoon naps.

Sleeps about 8 hours daily. To bed at 11:00pm up at 7:30am. No difficulty falling asleep, does not use medication to sleep, no nightmares. Feels rested upon awakening.

Health has been "status quo" since CABG in 1975; at present she is worried that graft is blocked and more surgery will be required. Follows doctor's therapeutic regimen, and in order to keep healthy she eats foods from 4 basic food groups; does not smoke and does not drink alcoholic beverages; exercises moderately as arthritis permits.

Home is two stories with 8 rooms and she has been able

to do her own housework since recovery from CABG. Is very concerned that she will now need help with house cleaning. Her children see to the home repairs.

Receiving
Patient is fairly satisfied with herself and proud that she has been independent ever since the death of her husband. Says help from her children is welcome but she never has to ask for it. Admits to feeling overwhelmed by her present illness.

Exchanging
Has been non-insulin-dependent diabetic since 1968, on low-fat 1000 cal diet and Diabinese qd.

Typical meal

Breakfast	oatmeal with milk, decaffeinated coffee— 1 cup
Lunch	cheese sandwich, orange, coffee
Dinner	beef patty, onions and mushrooms, melon or other fruit, 1 glass milk
PM Snack	3 vanilla wafer cookies

Takes no dietary supplements, drinks 6–7 glasses of fluid daily. Has gained 31 lbs since March 1984; present weight 156 lbs, ht. 4'10-1/2". Feels she follows diet in spite of admitted weight gain.

Note
At the end of the Health History and prior to the Physical Examination, several diagnoses can be formulated. More nursing diagnoses will be added following the Physical Examination.

At this point, the following nursing diagnoses should be considered:

Anxiety
Powerlessness

Alteration in nutrition: more than body requirements
Potential impaired home maintenance
Potential activity intolerance
Impaired skin integrity (to be validated in PE)

2 | Introduction to Routine Physical Examination

Before beginning the outline of the portions of the physical examination, several points should be emphasized. The physical examination is the systematic assessment of the physical and mental status of the patient and is considered objective data. During the physical examination, the patient is examined in a *series of steps* starting at the head and generally moving down the body. The approach is intended to gather as much information as possible on function, size, and appearance of organs and body parts in order to make a comprehensive and integrated evaluation of the presence or absence of pathology and the total body response to pathological processes.

A complete health history should be done before any part of the physical examination is performed. The exceptions are, of course, emergency situations or when the patient exhibits extreme pain, shortness of breath or other symptoms making a health history impossible. The major purpose of a good health history is to give the examiner clues as to physical problems that should be explored and verified in the physical examination. There are aspects of the patient's illness that are revealed only by physical examination. For these reasons, it is important that the physical examination be done thoroughly, skillfully, and in a logical sequence.

The four classical techniques of the physical examination are inspection, palpation, percussion, and auscultation. Each technique is performed separately and in sequence. A brief explanation of each technique includes:

Inspection
The visual examination of the body to detect significant physical findings. Inspection is more than just looking. It is a deliberate, systematic, and focused technique. It involves the discernment of what is normal, what deviates from normal but is within normal limits, and what is abnormal, requiring further attention.

Palpation
Examination of the body through the sense of touch to determine the characteristics of tissues and organs. Palpation involves not only the sense of touch but also the sense of temperature and the perception of movement, position, consistency and form.

Percussion
Examination of the body by tapping lightly but sharply on the body surface to produce sounds that reflect position, shape, size, and density of underlying organs and tissues. In most cases percussion is performed by placing the passive hand flat and holding it firmly against the area to be percussed, and striking the tip of pleximeter (middle) finger with the tip of the middle finger of the other hand. Percussion reflects the nature of the body cavities and is both heard and felt by the examiner. Percussion may also be used to determine areas of pain.

Auscultation
Listening through the use of a stethoscope to sounds produced in the body to assess normal or deviations from normal. Auscultation is useful in appraising sounds from the lungs, heart, stomach, intestines and from bruits or murmurs in the neck and abdomen.

These four techniques will be used when appropriate during each portion of the physical examination.

Equipment needed for a physical examination includes:

Scale with height attachment

Sphygmomanometer with appropriate size cuff
Stethoscope with diaphragm and bell
Ophthalmoscope/otoscope (pneumatic attachment for children)
Snellen Eye Chart
Tuning fork (500–1000 Hz for auditory screening
                     100–400 Hz for neuro exam)
Reflex hammer
Cotton balls
Safety pin
Tape measure
Flashlight or penlight
Latex gloves (several pairs)
Lubricant
If female: Vaginal speculum
                 Lubricant
                 Latex gloves
                 Pap smear equipment, if necessary
                 Adjustable light source

General Survey

Following the health history, a general survey statement is made. The general survey is a statement of the general impression of the "patient-as-a-whole." This initial survey is considered a scanning procedure, beginning with the first encounter with the patient and continuing during the health history. Major areas included in the general survey statement are the patient's mental status and level of consciousness, body development, nutritional state, speech, chronological versus apparent age, stature, and the character of the patient's general condition, such as presence of pain, shortness of breath, restlessness, tremors. Vital signs, height and weight may also be included in the general survey statement.

A sample of the general survey statement:

This is a 47-year-old alert, well-developed, well-nourished man who appears his chronological age and is in no acute distress. B/P 138/84, P88, R18. Dress and manner are appropriate. No apparent distinguishing body features. Speech is normal rate revealing intelligent thought pattern. Attentive with good body position and eye contact during interview. Weight seems appropriate for body build and height.

3 | Assessment of the Skin and Nails

SKIN

History Questions

Rash
  Description, location, onset, progression; accompanying symptoms such as itching, pain; allergies to environment, drugs or food; seasonal or occupational relationship; exposure to contagious skin conditions
Lesions
  Description, location, onset; accompanying symptoms such as itching, pain
  Recent color changes
    Vitiligo, hyperpigmentation, jaundice
Recent diagnosis of immunological disorders (deficiency) accompanied by appearance of nodular cutaneous lesions
Change in moles
  Color, shape, size, sensitivity, itching
Vascular changes
  Petechiae, ecchymosis, bruising, spider angioma
Family history
  Allergic, acute, intermittent, or chronic problems
Psychological response
  Withdrawal from social activities; cosmetics; change in self-image

Previous treatment
Change in nails
Color, shape, size, edges, thickness, angle

Examination

The techniques of inspection and palpation are used principally in examination of the skin. The fingertips are sensitive to fine tactile detail and are therefore best suited to palpating lesions and masses; the thin dorsal aspects of the fingers or hands are best suited to palpating skin temperature.

Inspection and Palpation

Inspect and palpate general overall and specific skin areas beginning with hands, forearms, and face and continuing throughout the physical examination.
Note:

Color: Pallor, flushing, cyanosis, redness, brownness, jaundice
Vascularity: Dilated superficial veins, evidence of bleeding or bruising, petechiae, ecchymosis
Temperature: Feel skin to assess increased local warmth or coolness.
Texture: Roughness, smoothness, thickness
Moisture: Dryness, sweating, oiliness
Mobility and turgor: Ease with which the skin moves (mobility) and returns to place (turgor)

In dehydration, senile cutaneous atrophy, or rapid loss of body fluid, skin turgor is diminished. Loss of turgor is evident when the skin remains in a fold after pinching. This is referred to as "tenting."
Lesions should be described in the following manner:

Color
Size
Configuration (diffuse, discrete, well circumscribed)

Shape consistency (soft, hard)
Odor
Effect of pressure
Pulsatility
Distribution over body—localized or generalized—on exposed skin surface or skin folds
Arrangement (clustered, linear, annular, or dermatomal)
Relationship to hair follicle
Primary and/or secondary lesions
> Primary lesions develop without any preceding skin changes
>
> Secondary lesions result from changes in primary lesions and are influenced by scratching, infection, and treatment

Mobility

(See Figure 3–1 and Tables 3–1 and 3–2.)

Skin conditions in persons with dark skin may be difficult to assess. Examine dark skin using the considerations outlined in Table 3–3.

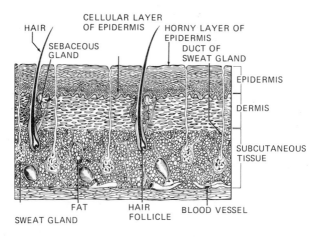

Figure 3–1. Anatomy of the skin.

TABLE 3-1. PRIMARY SKIN LESIONS

Lesion	Description	Example	
Macule	Change in skin color Less than 1 cm No change in consistency or elevation of skin Can be caused by inflammatory dilation of small blood vessels Not palpable	Freckles Flat moles Rubella Drug eruptions First degree burns Lupus erythematosus	
Papule	Circumscribed *solid* elevation Not over 1 cm	Lichen Planus Some warts Acne Insect bites Psoriasis	
Nodule	Increased elevation or consistency over papule 1-2 cm Can be soft or hard	Nodulus Cutaneous Pigmented nevi Gummas Xanthomas	

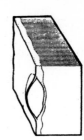
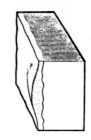

Tumor

Solid mass
Over 2 cm

Dermatofibroma
Epithelioma

Wheal

Fluid held diffusely in tissue,
temporarily raising skin
(contains no blood or free fluid)
1 mm to several cm

Urticaria
Mosquito bites

Vesicle or Bulla

Circumscribed elevation
Serous fluid flows easily if wall is
punctured
Vesicle: less than 1 cm
Bulla: more than 1 cm

Vesicle: blisters, cold
sores, chicken pox
Bulla: pemphigus

(continued)

TABLE 3-1. PRIMARY SKIN LESIONS (Continued)

Lesion	Description	Example
Pustule	Vesicle or bulla with fluid discolored by mixture of white cells, cellular debris, microorganisms 1 mm to 1 cm (lesions with larger amounts of pus are referred to as furuncles, abscesses, or carbuncles)	Acne vulgaris Impetigo

TABLE 3-2. SECONDARY SKIN LESIONS

Lesions	Description	Example
Crust	Thickened, dried-out fluid From serous fluid, purulent infection or blood oozing	Impetigo Eczema
Plaque	Lesion resulting from coalescence of wheals Large elevated plateau-like lesion	Hives
Pustule	Infected papule (may also be primary)	Acne

(continued)

TABLE 3-2. SECONDARY SKIN LESIONS (Continued)

Lesions	Description	Example
Scale	Excess of horny material on skin's surface Flakes of skin	Pityriasis rosea Psoriasis
Fissure	Linear break in epidermis Crack in skin surface Erosion (scoop out break in epidermis; no scarring)	Eczema Chapping

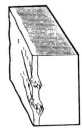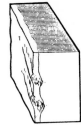

Ulcer — Deeper break in epidermis; may extend deeply into corium and subcutaneous tissue; may scar — Chancre, Stasis ulcer

Scar — Skin repaired with fibrous tissue or excess collagen — Postoperative scar, Keloid

TABLE 3-3. EXAMINATION OF DARK SKIN

Condition	Consideration
Petechiae	Usually appear in mucous membranes in diseases manifesting petechiae
	Inspect buccal mucosa and the bulbar and palpebral conjunctiva
Erythema	Associated with rash; palpate for papular type lesion
	From carbon monoxide poisoning and polycythemias; observe lips
Ecchymosis	Differentiate from erythema; pressure on skin causes erythema to blanch
	Inspect buccal mucosa and the conjunctivae
Pallor (absence of underlying red tones which give dark skin a glow)	Will appear yellowish brown or ashen gray
	Inspect mucous membrane, lips, and nail beds
Cyanosis	Need to be familiar with person's precyanotic state
	Inspect lips, nails, ear lobes, palpebral conjunctiva
	Apply pressure on tissue, color returns normally in less than 1 second
	In cyanosis, color returns by spreading more slowly from periphery to center of area where pressure applied
Jaundice	Inspect sclera when eyelids are in regular visual position. Can be confused with pigmentation (some persons normally have subconjunctival fat with carotene, which becomes darker farther from cornea)
	If yellowish near cornea, jaundice may be present

TABLE 3-4. ABNORMALITIES OR VARIATIONS OF NAILS

Abnormality or Variation	Cause
Badly mutilated, bitten	Usually nervous habit of biting
Beau's line	Matrix forms transverse indentation during severe illness
Clubbing: Early, Late	Often associated with cardiac or respiratory disorders. Early clubbing can be detected by noting whether or not the normal slight angle is present between the nail and finger and if the nailbed is soft and spongy; in late clubbing the fingertips become wider and rounder; the overlying skin stretches, with a polished, glistening appearance

Early

Late

(continued)

TABLE 3–4. ABNORMALITIES OR VARIATIONS OF NAILS (Continued)

Abnormality or Variation	Cause
Splinter hemorrhages	Thin, brownish, flame-shaped lines in the nail bed. Occurs with minor trauma, emboli from subacute bacterial endocarditis or without specific cause
Red half-moons in nail bed	Cardiac failure
Subungual hematoma	Blow to nail

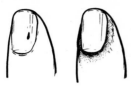

Subungual glomus tumor   Growth under nail

Paronychia   Inflammed skin around nail

From Lehrer, S. *Understanding Lung Sounds*. W.B. Saunders Co., Philadelphia: 1984. Used with permission of publisher.

TABLE 3-5. SKIN LESIONS: VASCULAR AND NEOPLASTIC

Lesions	Description	Examples
Vascular		
Telangiectasia	Fine red streaks due to dilated blood vessels (venules, capillaries, arterioles)	Appear on alae nasae of most adults. May occur at any age in both sexes anywhere on skin or mucous membranes. Normal finding
Spider angiomas	Cutaneous lesions with a central red pulsating arteriole; small fine vessels radiate from this like the legs of a spider	Frequently found in chronic liver disease. May occur in normal individuals and during pregnancy
Petechiae	Tiny reddish-brown capillary hemorrhages, 0.50 mm in diameter, found within skin papillae, due to capillary fragility	Patients with vitamin deficiency, blood dyscrasias, severe infections
Ecchymoses	Larger hemorrhages or bruises under the skin, several millimeters to several centimeters in size	Patients with blood dyscrasias or trauma

Neoplastic

Kaposi's sarcoma	Cutaneous nodules affecting skin of distal lower extremities. Skin between nodules may be edematous with malformed dilated vessels	Elderly patients may have this manifestation
Kaposi's sarcoma related to immune suppression	Multicentric, pigmented, painless, non-pruritic cutaneous lesions that may extend to many body sites including lymphatic and nodular involvement	Relatively confined to HIV-positive patients
In immune suppressed disease Kaposi's Sarcoma—Non-HIV-positive	Cutaneous nodules primarily affecting skin of distal extremities. Skin between the nodules may be edematous with malformed dilated vessels	Elderly patients may have this manifestation
Kaposi's sarcoma HIV-positive	Multicentric, pigmented, painless, non-pruritic cutaneous lesions that may extend to any body site and include lymphatic and nodule involvement	Relatively confined to male homosexual
Basal cell epithelioma	Translucent nodule that spreads, leaving a depressed center and firm, elevated border. Grows slowly and rarely metastasizes	Common on the face of fair-skinned adults over 40

(continued)

TABLE 3–5. SKIN LESIONS: VASCULAR AND NEOPLASTIC (Continued)

Lesions	Description	Examples
Squamous cell carcinoma	Found usually on the face and back of hands of sun-exposed skin; an actinic keratosis, usually firmer and redder than basal cell epithelioma	Common in fair-skinned adults over 60
Malignant melanoma	Change in growth or color of a benign mole; color varies; lesion is raised with a surface that is irregular, ulcerated and crusted. Highly malignant	Common in fair-skinned individuals

NAILS

Inspection and Palpation
Inspect and palpate the fingernails and toenails for consistency noting color, shape, lesions, general condition (Tables 3–4 and 3–5.)

Recording

Normal
Skin is pink, warm to the touch with good moisture, texture, and turgor without excoriations or lesions. Nails are of uniform thickness without deformity; nail beds pink with no apparent clubbing.

Abnormal
Skin is pink and warm to touch with decreased mobility and turgor. Macular, papular, annular rash visible on chest, shoulders, and distal extremities. Nail edges are ragged with transverse depressions and irregular thickening. No lymphadenopathy.

The patient with these abnormal findings would be at high risk for the following nursing diagnoses:

Impaired skin integrity
Potential fluid volume deficit

4 | Assessment of the Head and Neck

History Questions

Headache
  Quality, location, severity, visual disturbance, nausea,
    vomiting, syncope, vertigo
  Radiation to neck and shoulders
  Migraine
  Provocative or palliative factors, i.e., position of head
  History of hypertension
  Medication
Past Injuries
  Severity, treatment, residual
Any noticeable changes
  Hair texture and amount
  Facial sensation, symmetry
  Facial skin texture and moisture

Examination

Inspection and Palpation
Inspect and palpate:

  Hair
    If wig is worn, remove for hair and skull examination
    Quality, distribution, texture, pattern of loss
    Differentiate between nits and dandruff

Scalp
    Hygiene, lumps, lesions
Skull
    General size and contour, deformities, depressions, lumps, or presence of underlying tenderness
Skin
    Color, pigmentation, texture, lesions, hair distribution
Face
    Facial expression and symmetry, areas of anesthesia or differences in touch sensation

Tables 4–1, 4–2, and 4–3 list various characteristics that may be signs of particular conditions.

NECK

History Questions

Lumps in neck, hoarseness, swelling
Difficulty swallowing
Swollen glands, difficulty or pain on biting
    or chewing
Frequent stiffness, arthritis, muscular weakness

TABLE 4-1. SKULL CHARACTERISTICS THAT MAY BE SIGNS OF PARTICULAR CONDITIONS

Characteristic	Condition
Abnormally small head	Associated with mental retardation
Abnormally large head	Associated with hydrocephalus or acromegaly
Abnormally elongated skull	Sometimes seen in sickle cell anemia

TABLE 4-2. HAIR CHARACTERISTICS THAT MAY BE SIGNS OF PARTICULAR CONDITIONS

Characteristics	Condition
Dryness, brittleness	Myxedema, aging
Fine, silky	Hyperthyroidism
Alopecia	Secondary syphilis
	Severe emotional stress
	Cytotoxic drugs for treatment of malignancy
Smooth, round lesions attached to overlying skin	Sebaceous cyst or wen
Crusts and flakes	Eczema, seborrheic dermatitis, dandruff, psoriasis
	Contact dermatitis from hair dye or spray

Enlarged thyroid
Pain
Changes in range of motion (ROM) of cervical spine

Examination

Inspection
Inspect for symmetry, masses, scars, normal cervical concavity of cervical spine. Ask the patient to perform range of motion of the neck including flexion, hyperextension, lateral flexion, and rotation. Inspect trachea for any deviation from midline and difficulty swallowing and for venous jugular distention. (Figures 4–1 and 4–2 show anatomy of the head and neck.)

Palpation
Palpate the 10 lymph nodes in sequence.

Preauricular
Postauricular

TABLE 4-3. FACIAL SKIN CHARACTERISTICS AND EXPRESSIONS THAT MAY BE SIGNS OF PARTICULAR CONDITIONS

Expression	Condition
Grotesque, grinning expression due to spasm of facial muscles	Tetanus
Flat, expressionless, masklike faces with occasional drooling	Paralysis agitans (Parkinsonism)
Velvety smooth skin, wide-eyed, startled expression	Hyperthyroidism (with exophthalmus)
Faintly confused or quizzical expression	Deafness
Perpetual frown or squint	Poor vision
Expression of exhaustion or defeat	Malignant and chronic wasting disease, depression
Asymmetry of facial structures	Paresis or paralysis of facial muscles; Bell's palsy
Elevations of the skin surface over the nose, lips, cheeks, forehead or temple	Lipomas and basal cell or squamous cell carcinoma
Coarse, thickened facial skin that may produce a dull, sleepy expression, orbital edema	Hypothyroidism
Enlargement of bone and soft tissues. Elongated head with bony prominences of the forehead, nose, and lower jaw	Acromegaly
Round or "moon" face with red cheeks and excessive hair growth on the sideburn areas and on the chin	Cushing's syndrome

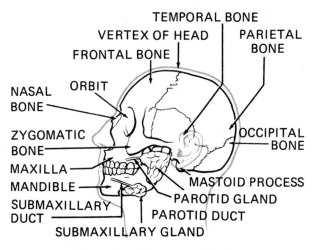

Figure 4–1. Lateral view of skull.

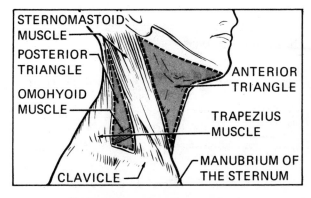

Figure 4–2. Anatomy of neck muscles.

Occipital
Parotid
Submaxillary
Submental
Superficial cervical
Posterior cervical
Deep cervical chain
Supraclavicular
Note: Size, shape, mobility, consistency, and tenderness
   of nodes (Figures 4–3 and 4–4).
Palpate *tempomandibular joint.*

Place tip of index finger in front of tragus of each ear and
ask the patient to open the mouth. Observe range of motion,
any swelling, or tenderness. Crepitus may be felt and heard,
which may be normal.

Palpate *trachea* to determine proper alignment (Figure
4–5).

Place finger over the trachea in the area of the sternal
notch. The trachea should be far enough posterior to allow a
fingertip to be inserted.

Palpate *thyroid* to determine size, shape, symmetry, tenderness, nodules. Rest your thumbs on the nape of the

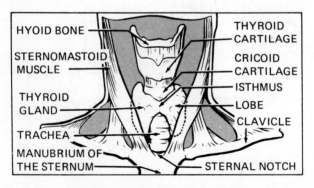

Figure 4–3. Internal anatomy of neck.

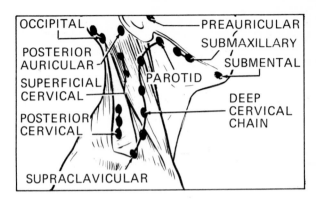

Figure 4–4. The lymph nodes of the head and neck.

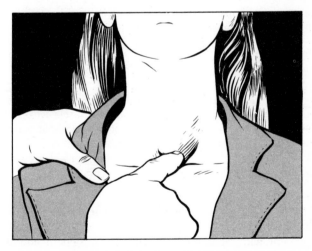

Figure 4–5. Palpation of the trachea.

patient's neck and with the index and middle fingers of both hands feel for the thyroid isthmus and for the anterior surfaces of the lateral lobes as patient swallows. The thyroid will move past the fingertip (upward) on swallowing (Figure 4–6A,B).

Palpate *carotid arteries* and *jugular veins*. Note rhythm, volume, equality of sides. Palpate carotid arteries by placing fingers medial to the sternomastoid muscle just below the jaw. Palpate only one side at a time to avoid carotid sinus massage (Figure 4–7).

Jugular veins of the neck may be distended or full in the recumbent position, but distention should not be visible at 45°. If distention or engorgement of the internal jugular vein is evident at 45°, the patient should be placed in a full upright position to see at what angle distention will diminish. Distention at any angle from 45° (Fowler's position) to 90° (upright) indicates venous obstruction or right heart failure.

Auscultation

Auscultate carotid pulses for rhythm, volume, weakness, bruits, or radiation of murmurs. If thyroid gland is enlarged to palpation, it should be auscultated with the diaphragm of the stethoscope for presence of a bruit.

Recording

Normal

Normocephalic with hair of fine texture and normal distribution. Face symmetrical with no apparent muscle weakness; sensation of touch intact. Full ROM of neck without venous distention or pulsation; carotid pulsations equal and of good quality bilaterally without bruits. Thyroid not enlarged and trachea midline. No lymphadenopathy.

Abnormal

At rest, face appears symmetrical with skin moderately dry to the touch. Upon speaking, asymmetry of face is readily apparent with right forehead and cheek smooth and not responding with the left side. Right lower eyelid sagging and

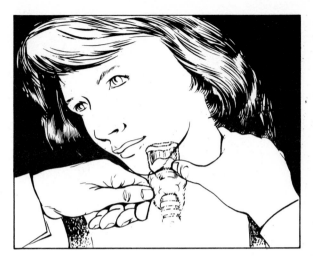

Figure 4–6A. Palpation of thyroid from front.

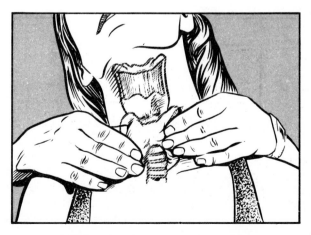

Figure 4–6B. Palpation of thyroid from behind.

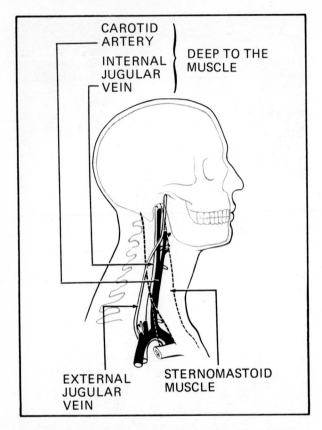

Figure 4–7. Jugular veins and carotid artery of the neck.

right corner of mouth drooping. Unable to clench jaw or show teeth on right side. Sensation to face intact bilaterally. Carotid pulsations equal bilaterally; trachea midline. No lymphadenopathy.

The patient with these abnormal findings would be at high risk for the following nursing diagnosis:

Body image disturbance

5 | Assessment of the Mouth and Pharynx

History Questions

Lesions or soreness of mouth or tongue
  Onset, cause, treatment
Difficulty with gums
  Bleeding, recession, pain
Change in color of lips
Previous surgery
  Gums, mouth
Voice changes
  Onset, duration, treatment
Difficulty swallowing
Sore throat
  Frequency, treatment
Teeth
  Caries, dentures, partial plate

Examination

Inspection
Inspect the mouth and throat in the following order:

Lips for color, moisture, lumps, ulcer, cracking, ulcerative lesions, symmetry.
Buccal mucosa and parotid duct orifice for color, pigmentation, ulcer, nodules.

Gums for inflammation, swelling, bleeding, retraction, hypertrophy, or discoloration.

Teeth for looseness, caries, partial plate, abnormal position, biting, chewing surface.

Roof of mouth for color, architecture of hard palate (remove dentures for inspection).

Tongue for color, papillae, abnormal smoothness, midline, presence of lesions.

Pharynx for anterior and posterior pillars, uvula; tonsils for color, symmetry, enlargement, exudate; posterior pharynx.

Palpation

With gloved hand, palpate lesion of the lip or buccal mucosa, floor of the mouth and tongue to detect masses or tenderness.

Recording

Normal

Lips moist and pink. Buccal mucosa and gingiva pink and moist without plaques or lesions. Soft and hard palate intact. Teeth in good repair with many fillings visible. Tongue protrudes in midline without deviation or fasiculations. Uvula rises midline. Tonsil tags present with no redness.

Abnormal

Lips, buccal mucosa, and gingiva pink and moist without plaques or lesions. Softening, fissuring, and cracking at angles of mouth bilaterally. Soft and hard palate intact without irritation. Poorly fitting dentures negate clear speech and proper handling of saliva (Figures 5–1 and 5–2).

The patient with these abnormal findings would be at high risk for the following nursing diagnosis:

Body image disturbance

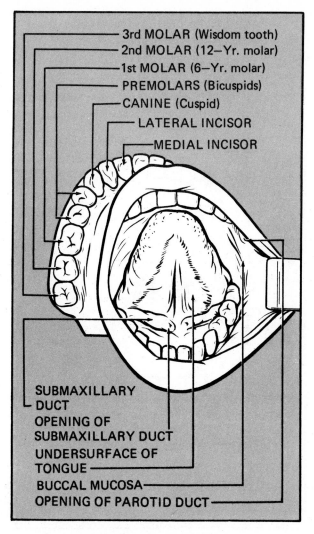

Figure 5–1. Structures of the mouth.

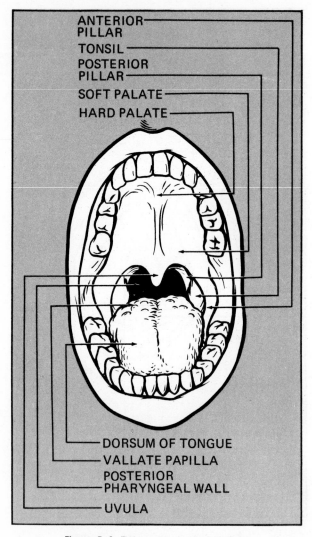

Figure 5–2. The mouth and the pharynx.

6 | Assessment of the Nose and Sinuses

History Questions

Nasal discharge
   Known allergies, epistaxis
Ability to smell
   Stuffiness, polyps
   Use of cocaine
Frequency and description of respiratory conditions
   Allergic rhinitis, postnasal drip
   Medication
Related surgery
   T&A, deviated septum
Frequent headaches

Examination

Inspection
Inspect nose for deformity, asymmetry, inflammation. Inspect nasal mucosa for color, moisture, swelling, bleeding, ulceration, exudate of mucosa. Inspect nasal septum for deviation, perforation, bleeding, or ulceration. Inspect inferior turbinates and possibly middle turbinates for color, moisture, exudate, polyps.

Palpation
Palpate frontal and maxillary sinuses for soreness or tenderness. Transilluminate sinuses.

Recording

Normal
Nasal mucosa pink. No septal deviation or perforation; nares patent bilaterally with sense of smell intact. No sinus tenderness.

Abnormal
Nasal mucosa bright red bilaterally with swelling and mucopurulent exudate present. Unable to visualize turbinates. Extreme left frontal and maxillary sinus tenderness (Figures 6–1, 6–2, and 6–3).

The patient with these abnormal findings would be at high risk for the following nursing diagnoses:

Infection
Pain

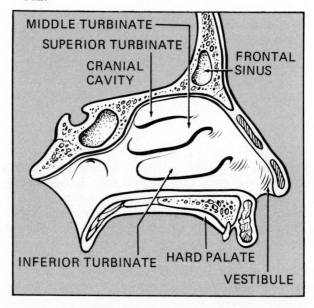

Figure 6–1. Left nasal cavity.

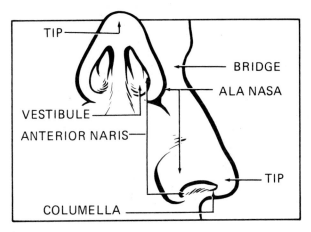

Figure 6–2. External anatomy of the nose.

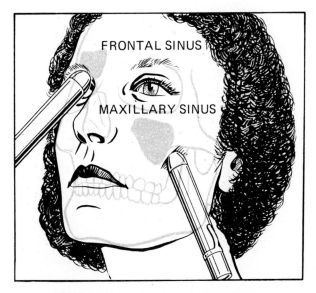

Figure 6–3. Transillumination of sinus cavities.

7 | Assessment of the Eye

History Questions

Difficulty with vision
  Blurring with near objects, with far objects, photophobia, diplopia
  Night blindness, halo around lights
Evidence of eye fatigue
  Tiredness, headaches
Inflammation
  Hyperemia, itching, burning, tearing, pain
Known problems
  Cornea, iris, nystagmus, strabismus, hordeolum, chalazion
Date of last eye exam
Current corrective lenses
Use of contact lenses
  Soft, hard, or extended wear
  Care of contact lenses

Examination
Perform tests for:

Visual Acuity
  Snellen chart for distance vision
  Pocket card or newsprint for near vision
Visual Fields

Gross confrontation of the visual fields is tested by comparing the patient's peripheral vision with the examiner's vision (assuming normal vision of examiner). With examiner and patient facing each other, one eye is covered and the examiner brings a wiggling finger into the visual fields until it is seen by the patient. This is repeated for each visual field and for each eye. Note any visual field deficits.

Corneal Light Reflex

Determine symmetrical or asymmetrical position of light reflections on the right and left eyes.

External Eye Inspection (See Table 7–1 for common abnormalities of the external eye.)

Inspect the eye, its orbit and surrounding tissue.

Eyebrows for distribution, position, alignment and movement.

Eyelashes for distribution, color, texture, and position.

Eyelids for color, edema, mobility, superficial vascularity, position-alignment.

Lacrimal apparatus for edema tenderness and redness.

Orbit for forward or backward displacement of the eye in its socket and alignment.

Conjunctiva for color, injection, moisture, lesions.

Sclera for color.

Cornea for smoothness, clarity, corneal reflex.

Iris for color and pattern.

Pupillary Examination

Examine pupil for equality, shape, pupillary constriction both direct and consensual; accommodation, and covergence, by use of penlight. May record as PERRLA (pupils equal, react to light and accommodate)

TABLE 7-1. ABNORMALITIES OF THE EXTERNAL EYE

Name	Definition	Physical Characteristics
Ectropian	The abnormal outward turning of the margin of the eyelid	The palpebral conjunctiva is exposed; the punctum of the lower lid turns outward, interfering with normal eye drainage producing excessive tearing. Infection may occur. Often found in the elderly
Entropian	The abnormal inward turning of the margin of the eyelid	The inward turned lashes, which may appear invisible, often produce irritation of the conjunctiva and cornea. Also occurs often in the elderly
Ptosis	The drooping of the upper eyelid	The affected lid almost covers the upper portion of the iris and part of the pupil. Unilateral or bilateral ptosis usually results from innervation or lid muscle disorder
Hordeolum (STY)	Infection of a sebaceous gland at the margin of the eyelid	A pustule is found on the lid margin often surrounded by hyperemia and swelling. Usually it will rupture and heal spontaneously

(continued)

TABLE 7-1. ABNORMALITIES OF THE EXTERNAL EYE (Continued)

Name	Definition	Physical Characteristics
Chalazion	Acute inflammation and obstruction of a meibomian gland	A small localized swelling of the eyelid that frequently causes a protrusion of the lid. Eversion of the lid shows hyperemia and an enlarged gland
Xanthelasma	Slightly raised, yellow, well circumscribed plaques in the skin appearing along the nasal portion of one or both eyelids	Plaques may occur on the upper or lower lids. Growth is slow and they may disappear spontaneously. Frequently associated with hypercholesteremia
Exophthalmous	The abnormal protrusion of the eyeball	Eyeball protrudes beyond the supra-orbital ridge of the frontal bone. Edema of the upper and lower lids with severe conjunctivitis may be present. Bilateral ophthalmous is suggestive of thyrotoxicosis; unilateral suggests a tumor or inflammation within the orbit

| Enophthalmous | The abnormal backward placement of the eyeball | The eyeball is recessed in the orbit. When bilateral the cause is usually dehydration; when unilateral trauma or inflammation is suspected |
| Dacrocystitis | Inflammation of the lacrimal sac | There is swelling between the lower eyelid and nose from inflammation of the lacrimal sac. If acute, there is pain, redness and tenderness and/or surrounding cellulitis; if chronic, obstruction of the naso lacrimal duct is usually present. Excessive tearing occurs. By applying pressure to the lacrimal sac, fluid from the sac can be expressed via the punctae of the eyelid |

Palpation

Palpate the eyes gently. If abnormal eyeball tension is suspected, intraocular pressure is best measured by the tonometer. All persons over 40 years of age should be checked every two years by tonometry.

Extraocular Muscle Function

Perform test for extraocular movement (EOM). Check six cardinal positions of gaze.

Position	Muscle	Nerve
Horizontal temporal	Lateral rectus	Abducens VI
Up and temporal	Superior rectus	Oculomotor III
Down and temporal	Inferior rectus	Oculomotor III
Horizontal nasal	Medial rectus	Oculomotor III
Up and nasal	Inferior oblique	Oculomotor III
Down and nasal	Superior oblique	Trochlear IV

Ophthalmoscopic Examination

(Table 7–2 lists some abnormalities on ophthalmoscopy.)

Procedure/ Structure	Normal Characteristics	Abnormal Findings
Inspect *red reflex* for shape and color	Round and bright with red orange glow	Reflex has diminished color, dark spots, and irregular shape
Inspect *optic disc* for:		
Location	Located on the nasal side of the center of retina	Because of papilledema, there is swelling of the disc

Procedure/ Structure	Normal Characteristics	Abnormal Findings
		when the venous drainage of capillaries is impeded. Disc margins are blurred and appear to project forward
Shape	Round or vertically oval	Irregular shape with blurred margins
Color	Creamy pink or yellowish red, brighter than surrounding retina	Pallor of part or all of disc
Size	Approximately 1.5 mm; symmetrical in both eyes	Not equal in both eyes
Physiologic cup	Depression located toward temporal side of disc; lighter in color. Cup never extends to margins in normal fundus	Cup location and size are not symmetrical in both eyes
Inspect the retinal vessels for:		
Appearance	Arteries are lighter in color and smaller than veins; veins are	Veins are pale in color; arteries less than 3/5 size of veins

Procedure/ Structure	Normal Characteristics	Abnormal Findings
	darker in color and larger than arteries	
Distribution	Main artery and veins of eye enter and leave the optic nerve behind the disc. Vessels regular in shape and decrease in size as they branch and move toward the periphery	Irregularity of shape of vessels with uneven distribution
Inspect retinal background for appearance	Color is uniform but varies widely from person to person	Pallor of the fundus; soft or hard exudates
Inspect macula for appearance	The last structure to be assessed, it is seen as slightly darker than the retina and the same size of the optic disc. The fovea centralis is seen as a speck of light reflected from the center—the region of the retina with highest visual acuity	Pigment clumped; areas lacking in pigment

TABLE 7-2. SOME ABNORMALITIES ON OPHTHALMOSCOPY

Finding	Interpretation	Example	Figure
Pale white disc; pallor extends to disc margins; disc vessels absent	Death of optic nerve fibers	Optic atrophy	

Optic Atrophy

(continued)

TABLE 7-2. SOME ABNORMALITIES ON OPHTHALMOSCOPY (Continued)

Finding	Interpretation	Example	Figure
Disc margins blurred; physiologic cup not visible, disc appears to project forward (Papillaedema)	Venous stasis	Increased intracranial pressure Mass lesions Hypertension	 Papillaedema
Base of cup pale; cup enlarged and extends to edge of disc	Increased intraocular pressure	Glaucoma	 Glaucoma

	Thickening of the retinal arteriole	Aging Arteriosclerosis Hypertension
Arteries change color, become opaque, show copper wire or silver wire defect		 Silver Wire Defect
	Microaneurysms	Diabetic retinopathy
Tiny red spots commonly located in the macular area		 Diabetic Retinopathy

(continued)

TABLE 7-2. SOME ABNORMALITIES ON OPHTHALMOSCOPY (Continued)

Finding	Interpretation	Example	Figure
Vein stops abruptly or tapers on either side of arteriole	Arteriovenous nicking	Aging Arteriosclerosis With or without hypertension Retinal diseases	 AV Nicking
Streaked flame-shaped hemorrhages paralleling the blood vessels	Capillary insufficiency or ischemia	Hypertensive retinopathy	 Hypertensive Retinopathy

Cotton Wool Patches
(Soft Exudates)

Hard Exudates

Fluffy, white "soft" exudate (cotton wool patches)

Hypertensive changes of a terminal arteriole; thickening and swelling of the terminal retinal nerve fibers

Diabetes
Connective tissue disease
Hypertension
Papilledema

Round, yellowish-white deposits in retina (hard exudate)

Edema residues from leaking capillaries or arterioles or degenerating nerve tissue

Hypertension
Diabetes

Recording

Normal
Eyelashes and brows present bilaterally. Vision in right eye (OD) and left eye (OS) 20/20 using Snellen chart. Conjunctiva and sclera clear. Pupils equal, round, react to light and accommodate (PERRLA). Visual fields normal by confrontation. Extraocular movements (EOM) intact without nystagmus or strabismus. Red reflex present, disc margins sharp. No AV nicking, hemorrhages, or exudates. Macula normal. Foveal reflex present.

Abnormal
Eyelashes and brows present bilaterally. Normal ocular tension. Vision via Snellen chart is OD 20/20 and OS 20/40.

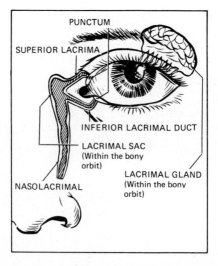

Figure 7–1. External anatomy of the eye.

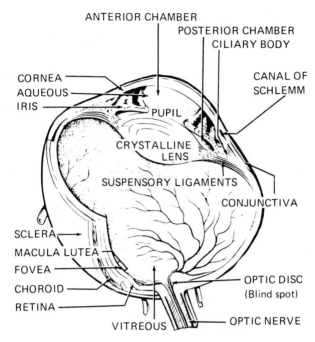

Figure 7-2. Anatomical structure of the eye.

Conjunctiva and sclera clear (PERRLA). EOM intact. Red reflex faint. Disc margin blurred. Hemorrhages visible in retina. Arteries narrow, tortuous with compression of veins.

The patient with these abnormal findings would be at high risk for the following nursing diagnosis:

Visual alterations
(See Figures 7-1 through 7-6.)

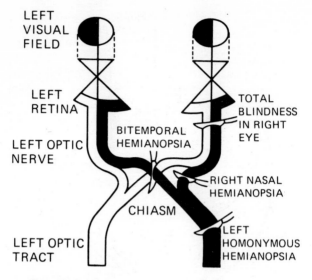

Figure 7–3. Schematic drawing of visual fields including visual field defects.

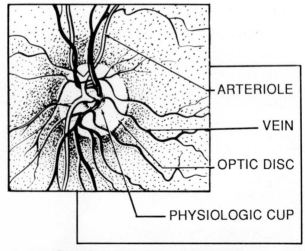

Figure 7–4. Optic disc and blood vessels.

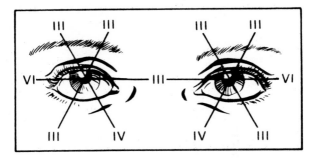

Figure 7–5. Cardinal positions of gaze.

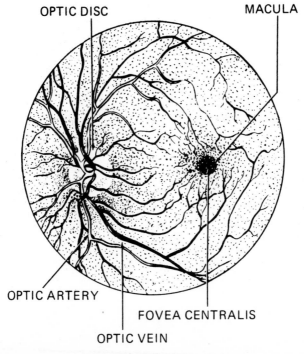

Figure 7–6. Fundus of the eye.

8 | Assessment of the Ear

History Questions

Difficulty hearing
  Recent changes, factor affecting this
  Hearing aid, type used, any problems
Pain in ear, vertigo, tinnitus
Discharge, past history of problems
Recent URI, allergies, sinusitis

Examination of External Ear

Inspection
Inspect both auricles for position, size, deformities, and symmetry. Observe the skin for color, lesions, or nodules. Finally, observe the external canal for evidence of any discharge.

Palpation
Palpate auricles for nodules, tophi, and tenderness by pulling on pinna and pushing on tragus. *Note:* Movements of pinna and tragus are generally very painful with external otitis and less so with otitis media (Figure 8–1).

Examination of Internal Ear
The internal ear is examined with the use of an otoscope, which provides an easily held intense light for illumination. The otoscope is held in one hand and the auricle is held by the

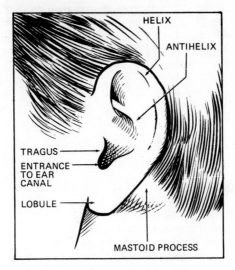

Figure 8–1. External anatomy of the ear.

thumb and index finger of the opposite hand (Figures 8–2 and 8–3).

Inspection

Examine the auditory canal as the otoscope is inserted. Pull the auricle upward and back in an adult and downward and back in a child to straighten the auditory canal and facilitate insertion.

Identify wax (cerumen), discharge, tumors or foreign bodies in ear canal. Identify tympanic membrane (TM) and landmarks. These landmarks include the manubrium and short process of the *malleus* the *umbo* or point at the center of the tympanic membrane where the malleus is attached, the *cone of light* or light reflex caused by reflection from otoscope light and the *annulus,* which is the outer edge of the ear drum and is usually lighter in color. Normal direction for cone of light reflection is toward the right in the right ear and toward the left in the left ear (Figures 8–4 and 8–5).

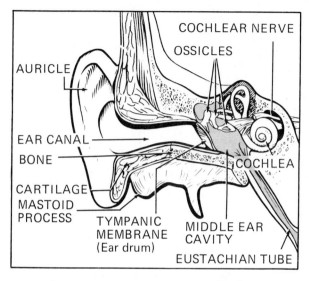

Figure 8–2. Internal anatomy of the ear.

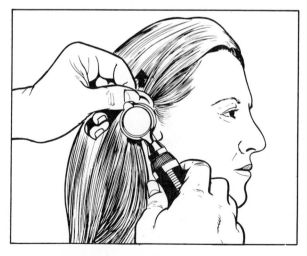

Figure 8–3. Ear position for otoscopy.

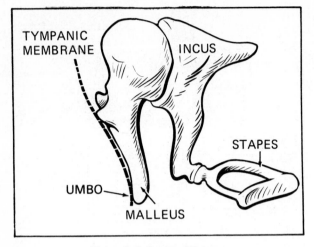

Figure 8–4. Bones of the ear.

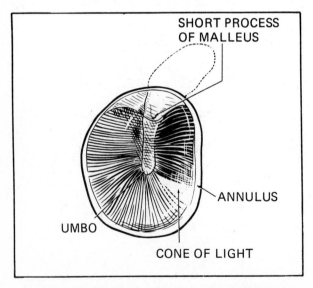

Figure 8–5. Landmarks of the tympanic membrane.

The speculum of the otoscope will need to be rotated anteriorially to see the entire drum. Note color and luster of TM, presence or absence of light reflex, and any lesions or abnormalities of TM. The most commonly seen abnormalities are white plaques or white flecks on the drum, indicating a healed inflammatory process and small, often misshapen black areas indicating a perforation of the drum (Table 8–1 lists abnormalities revealed on otoscopy).

Function—Hearing Test
There are several hearing tests that can be used to get a rough estimate of the patient's hearing acuity. All of these are merely

TABLE 8-1. SOME ABNORMALITIES ON OTOSCOPY

Finding	Interpretation	Examples
Bright red drum	Inflammation	Acute middle ear infection (otitis media)
Yellowish drum	Pus or serum behind drum	Acute or chronic otitis media
Bluish drum	Blood behind drum	Skull fracture
Hairline meniscus curve or bubbles behind drum	Serous fluid in middle ear	Acute serous otitis media or chronic otitis media
Absent light reflex, obscure landmarks	Bulging of drum	Acute otitis media
Absent or diminished landmarks	Thickening of drum	Chronic otitis media or otitis externa
Oval dark areas	Perforation	Recent or old rupture of drum
Malleus very prominent	Retraction of drum	Obstruction of Eustachian tube

From Sherman J, and Fields S: *Guide to Patient Evaluation.* Medical Examination Publishing Co., Inc., New York, 1978. Used with permission of the publisher.

screening tests and, if a hearing loss is identified, a more sophisticated audiometer examination is necessary to determine the degree and range of hearing loss present.

In a routine physical examination only one of these hearing tests needs to be done since any deficit will require further testing if treatment is indicated.

Whispered Voice Test

Because hearing the spoken word is the principal function of the auditory system, the level of voice needed for adequate hearing is perhaps the easiest and most useful test of hearing function. The examiner should already have a clue about any hearing difficulty from the patient response during the health history interview. For this test have patient occlude one ear at a time and, after making sure patient cannot read your lips, whisper clearly a phrase or several words until patient can repeat the words. Repeat procedure with both ears noting differences in perception between ears and level of voice needed for patient to hear (ie, soft whisper, loud whisper, normal voice, loud voice).

The following two tests require a tuning fork and will give information on whether the hearing loss is a conduction or perceptive (sensorineural) defect. In order to approximate the hearing range necessary for understanding spoken words, the tuning fork should be the 512 Hz or 1024 Hz frequency (human speech is roughly 500 to 2000 Hz). With sensorineural deafness, certain of the high pitches are lost whereas the lower tones are still perceived; therefore, the pitch of the tuning fork may influence the test (Figure 8–6).

Weber Test

Strike the tuning fork and, holding it by its stem, press firmly against skull in midline on top of head or on forehead. Ask patient in which ear sound is heard best. Sound should be heard equally well in both ears. A definite *lateralization* to one ear is abnormal.

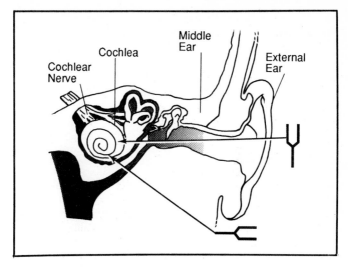

Figure 8–6. Pathways of air and bone conduction for hearing.

Rinne Test
Strike tuning fork and place stem on mastoid process behind ear until patient can no longer hear the sound. Then quickly place tuning fork near ear canal and check if sound can be heard. Normally, air conduction is better than bone conduction (AC>BC). Repeat with other ear and record findings.

	Weber Test	**Rinne Test**
Conduction loss	Lateralized to *poor* ear because poor ear is not distracted by room noise, sound perceived better in this ear.	BC>AC Normal conduction through ear blocked and bone vibrations bypass blockage.

	Weber Test	**Rinne Test**
Sensorineural loss (nerve loss)	Lateralized to *good* ear, nerve loss in poor ear unable to receive vibrations	AC>BC Normal pattern even in poor ear as nerve loss unable to receive vibrations by either route.

Function—Vestibular

Romberg. Have patient stand with feet together and eyes open. If patient does not begin to fall, have the patient close his or her eyes. With labyrinthine stimulation, the patient tends to fall in the direction of the flow of endolymph. Falling may also indicate neurological impairment. Be prepared to catch the patient when test is performed!

Recording

Normal
No lesions or masses of external ears or canals. No pain on palpation, no discharge, normal cerumen. TM pearly gray, landmarks visible, light reflex present bilaterally. Hears soft whisper easily bilaterally. Weber test equal bilaterally.

Abnormal
No lesions or masses of external ears or canals. Some pain on palpation of tragus of right ear. Right TM red, bulging, no landmarks or light reflex visible. Left TM pearly gray, landmarks visible, light reflex present. Whisper test shows evidence of diminished hearing in (R) ear; Weber test shows lateralization to (R) ear.

The patient with these abnormal findings would be at high risk for the following nursing diagnoses:

Pain
Altered auditory perception

9 | Assessment of the Breast and Axilla

History Questions

Self-examination
  When in menstrual cycle
  How often
Mammogram
  When, results
Lumps or masses in breast
  Past history and disposition
  Present condition, description, (size, location, mobility,
    pain, etc.), when first noticed, how discovered
Pain or tenderness in breast
  Description
  Relationship to menses
Discharge from nipples
  Description, onset
  Relationship to menses
Change in size of breast
  Relationship to menses
  Pregnancy or lactation
Pain in axilla
  Enlarged lymph nodes
  Rash or lesions

Examination

Patient Education

The most important part of this examination for female patients is teaching or reinforcing routine self-examination. Ask the patient, "Do you examine your breasts regularly? Please show me how you do it."

Inspection

Inspect for size, shape, symmetry (asymmetry not uncommon unless a *new* finding), supernumerary nipples, nipple retraction, dimpling, "orange peel" skin, venous pattern, lesions, ulcerations or discharge.

Have the patient perform the following maneuvers while in a sitting position and carefully observe for retractions or dimpling:

Raise hands above head

Clasp hands together in front of waist and push arms together forcefully to contract chest muscles, or place hands on posterior aspects of iliac crests and press down.

Inspect axilla and supraclavicular area for retractions, edema, or lesion.

Palpation

If patient has noted lump in breast, have her point it out, then palpate *opposite* breast first.

Palpate nipples and areolar area first to determine tenderness, nodules, or discharge.

Put patient supine with small pillow under scapula. Carefully palpate entire area of breast in an overlapping fashion being careful not to neglect tail of breast, which extends toward axilla. Pattern for palpation may be either quadrants or concentric circles; just make sure *all breast tissue is palpated* (Figures 9–1 through 9–3).

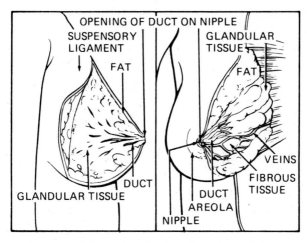

Figure 9–1. Internal and external anatomy of the breast.

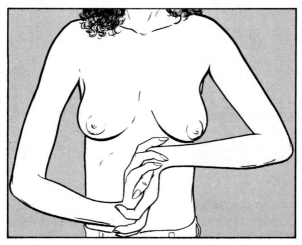

Figure 9–2. Contraction of pectoral muscles for breast exam.

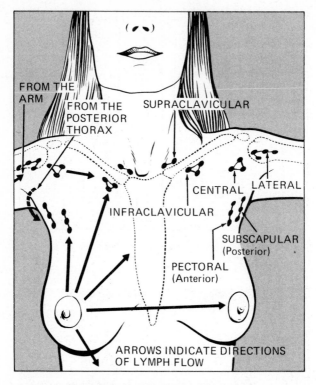

Figure 9–3. Lymph glands of the breast.

Palpate axillae, supra, and infraclavicular area for lymph nodes.

Masses should be described in the following manner:

Location (quadrant of breast; a sketch of location is helpful). Some people prefer to use a clock face in describing the location of a mass (eg, 6 o'clock, 2 cm from the nipple).

Size (cm)

Contour
Consistency
Mobility
Tenderness or pain
Other features (pulsation, color, accompanying features)

Special emphasis on self-breast examination should be given to women in high risk groups for breast cancer. These include:

Older than 50 years of age
History of:
> breast cancer in a close female relative (mother, sister, aunt, or grandmother), especially if the relative was premenopausal or had bilateral breast cancer
> previous breast cancer
> excessive exposure to ionizing radiation
> use of chemotherapy or other immunosuppressant drugs
> thymic atrophy and/or decreased number of thymus dependent lymphocytes
> nodular fibrocystic breasts
> oral contraceptive use particularly with a family history of breast cancer
> prolonged estrogen use between the ages of 10 and 12 and 42 and 55.
> cancer of the endometrium, ovary or colon

Birth of first baby after age 30
Early menarche and late menopause
Obesity with or without diabetes, wide body build
High intake or animal fats (a potential risk factor, although research is presently inconclusive)

Mammograms are low-dose radiographic studies of breast tissue and the recommendations by the American Cancer Society are:

Baseline mammogram between ages 35–39
Mammogram every 1–2 years for women ages 40–45
Mammogram every year for women over 45

Male Breast

The male breast should not be neglected, but does not require the special techniques of inspection described for the female patient. The male breast and axilla should be palpated in the same manner described for the female with the patient in a supine position. A pillow under the scapula is not necessary.

Breast of the Pregnant Female

In the pregnant female, breasts will increase in size as much as two to three times normal size in some patients. This enlargement may be accompanied by tenderness in the first trimester. The areolae and nipples become darker and the Montgomery's glands around the nipple area enlarge. Occasionally changes in the breasts will be the first sign of pregnancy a patient notices.

Nonmalignant Conditions of the Breast

Any change in the breast is certainly reason for concern, but the most common causes of signs and symptoms of breast disease are nonmalignant conditions.

Fibrocystic Breast Disease

This condition seems to be estrogen-related, as symptoms appear to be an exaggeration of the normal changes that occur in the breasts during the menstrual cycle, and the symptoms usually regress after menopause. The breast changes associated with fibrocystic disease advance from painful, tender breasts during menses to eventual formation of multiple cysts, which are usually bilateral, mobile, well delineated and tender premenstrually. The cysts are more common in the 30 to 55 age range and have been shown to disappear in some women when caffeine intake was eliminated. While diagnosis can be supported by clinical history, aspiration and biopsy are the best tools for a definitive diagnosis.

Adenofibroma

This is a benign tumor of the breast that occurs in women before the age of menopause. The mass is usually firm, well delineated, mobile, and nontender. A biopsy is recommended for a conclusive diagnosis, and in most cases the tumor is excised.

Other less common nonmalignant conditions of the breast include:

Mastitis
This is an inflammatory condition of the breasts, most common in nursing mothers. Breasts are very painful, hard, erythromatous; systemic symptoms of infection are also present.

Galactorrhea
This is nonpuerperal lactation and may be the result of various hormone imbalances (primarily prolactin) or drug ingestion.

Gynecomastia
This is the most common disorder of the male breast and is excessive development of the breast leading to a feminine appearance. In the majority of cases the condition is associated with a disturbance in the balance of estrogenic-androgenic effects on the mammary tissue. This finding may be associated with certain drugs including excessive use of marijuana, and with cirrhosis of the liver.

Recording

Normal
Right breast slightly larger than left. Contour and consistency appropriate for age and parity. No masses, lesions, or tenderness. Nipples with no retraction or discharge.

Abnormal
Symmetrical, moderate size. Right breast has firm, tender, oval mass 2 cm in diameter in upper outer quadrant approximately 3 cm from the nipple. Mass is mobile with no increased venous pattern or skin retraction. No discharge from (R) nipple. Left breast contour and consistency appropriate for age and parity, no masses or lesions. (L) nipple erect with no discharge.

The patient with these abnormal findings would be at high risk for the following nursing diagnoses:

Anxiety
Fear
Knowledge deficit

10 | Assessment of the Thorax and Lungs

History Questions

Cough
  How long, productivity, increasing frequency
Sputum
  Description and amount
Hemoptysis
  When, amount, frequency, description
Wheezing
  Onset, asthma, allergies, medications, precipitating factors
Shortness of breath
  When you first noticed it
  When it bothers you most
  How far you can walk or exercise, number of stairs
  How relieved
  Medications
Difficulty breathing at night
  Number of pillows to sleep, recent change
Pain in chest
  Description, onset, radiation, relief, medication
Last chest x-ray, results
Smoking
  How long
  Number of packs per day
Exposure to toxins and pollutants

Examination

Inspection

Inspect thorax for symmetry, size, shape, contour, and movement of chest. Observe respiratory pattern for puffed cheeks, use of accessory muscles, muscle retraction, or abnormal patterns such as:

Cheyne-Stokes Respirations. An irregular or cyclic pattern of breathing characterized by periods of apnea lasting 10–20 seconds.

Kussmaul Respirations. Characterized by deep, regular, sigh-like respirations. Rate may be fast, normal, or slow.

Stertorous Respirations. Snoring respirations, usually benign but may be caused by secretions in upper respiratory tract.

Stridulous Respirations. Characterized by high-pitched whistling or crowing sound. Heard in children with croup, foreign body in throat, diphtheria membrane, or growth in area of vocal chords.

Ataxic Respirations (Biot's breathing). Completely irregular, with some deep breaths followed by short shallow breaths. Rate is usually slow and may end in complete apnea.

Wheezing Respirations. Characterized by a prolonged expiratory time and often an audible wheeze or wheezes that can be heard on auscultation. Such respirations are typical of obstructive lung disease when air becomes trapped in the lungs.

Palpation and Percussion

Anterior Chest. Palpation of the anterior chest involves two steps. First, a general palpation of any areas of abnormalities to identify tenderness, masses, bony protrusions, crepitus (subcutaneous emphysema), or skin temperature changes. The second is to assess vocal fremitus. Fremitus is the vibration produced by the thoracic wall during phonation. The open palm of the hands should be placed on the chest wall and the patient asked to say "three" or "ninety-nine." Starting at the top of the chest wall and moving downward, the sides should be compared for differences in conduction. Normal vibrations made by breathing should not be felt. When fremitus is either increased or decreased on one side, particular note should be taken so that careful auscultation can further assess the problem. Vocal fremitus may be decreased in conditions such as pleural effusion, pleural thickening, pneumothorax, atelectasis, and emphysema. It may be increased when pulmonary consolidation occurs and alveoli are filled with fluid, thus increasing the sound transmission. This occurs also with lung masses and pulmonary fibrosis (Figures 10–1 and 10–2).

Next, percuss anterior chest in a systematic manner comparing sides as you progress from top to bottom of chest. Note excursion of diaphragm as patient inhales.

Percussion sounds in chest include:

Resonance: Air-filled lung tissue
Dullness: Less air-filled tissue, more solid tissue such as heart, liver, or lung consolidation
Flatness: No air in tissue, solid areas such as spine or pleural effusion
Tympany: Hollow, drum-like sound as over stomach area or large pneumothorax

Posterior Chest. Have patient flex head forward and cross arms at waist to separate scapulae. Palpate the posterior chest in a systematic manner, again noting any abnormalities. Palpate for vocal fremitus, noting any abnormalities. Voice sounds and tactile fremitus may be increased in the right lung field due to increased lung tissue on the right and possibly due to wider and straight right main bronchus. Finally, thoracic excursion or expansion is evaluated. To do this the thumbs are placed at the level of the 10th rib with the palms of the hands on the posteriolateral chest. The patient is asked to take a deep breath and the examiner observes for equal excursion of the rib cage.

Percuss posterior chest first with closed fist, starting at base of chest and moving toward shoulder to note any rib or muscle tenderness. Tenderness of the costovertebral angle is

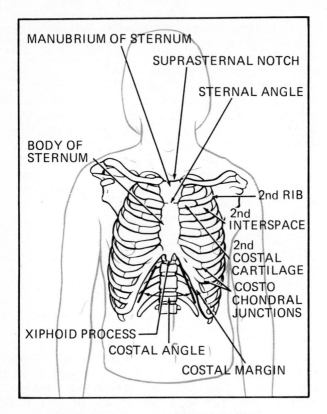

Figure 10–1. Anatomy of the anterior thorax.

termed "CVA tenderness," which may indicate kidney involvement.

Percuss posterior chest in usual manner, beginning at the top of the lungs and moving toward the base. Tables 10–1 and 10–2 list examples of chest and spinal deformities.

Generally the major assessment to be made with percussion of the posterior thorax is *diaphragmatic excursion,* the

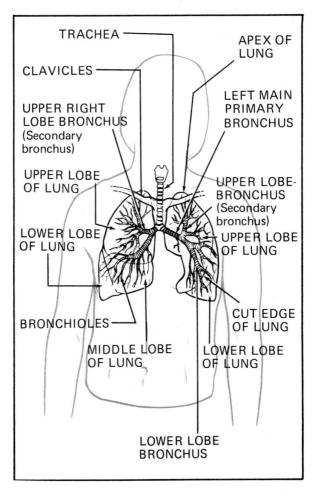

Figure 10–2. Anatomy of the respiratory system.

TABLE 10-1. CHEST DEFORMITIES

Chest Deformity	Description	Figure
Barrel chest	Increase in A/P diameter, sternum appears pulled forward, ribs more horizontal	
Pigeon breast or chicken breast	A/P diameter increased with transverse diameter narrowed vertical grooves in line of costochondral junctions	

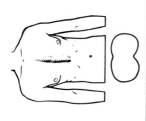

Pectus excavatum or
funnel chest

Ribs of lower part of sternum sink posteriorly
creating a pit (excavatum or funnel), this
decreases the A/P diameter

TABLE 10-2. SPINAL DEFORMITIES

Spinal Deformities	Description	Figure
Scoliosis (A)	Lateral curvature of the spin	
Kyphosis (B)	Increase in normal curvature of spine (hump back)	
Lordosis (C)	Concave curvature of spine	

distance the diaphragm lowers during full inspiration. The patient should be asked to inhale fully and the level of diaphragmatic dullness is noted. Next, the patient is asked to exhale fully and the level of the diaphragm is noted by percussion. Changes in resonant area due to diaphragm contraction (lowering) is usually 3–5 cm in females and 5–6 cm in males. This assessment is only a gross measurement, and any abnormal findings such as an abnormally high diaphragm level on one side suggesting pleural effusion should be followed up with a radiologic examination.

Auscultation

Auscultate anterior and posterior chest in a systematic manner comparing sides (Figure 10–3). Normal breath sounds (Figure 10–4) include vesicular, bronchial, and bronchovesicular. A description of these terms and a graphic illustration are shown below. Figure 10–5 shows the locations on the chest of these normal breath sounds.

Vesicular
  Normal, soft breath sounds
Bronchial
  Louder, tubular sounds, mostly during expiration. Heard at trachea and anterior chest of two main bronchi
Bronchovesicular
  Combination of vesicular and bronchial sounds. Heard in upper anterior chest and between scapulae on posterior chest
Tracheal
  Harsh blowing sound heard over trachea

Note: Deep breathing, especially with mouth open, will convert vesicular to bronchovesicular sounds. Soft moaning or grunting may be transmitted as abnormal breath sounds. Abnormal breath sounds are termed *adventitious sounds* and have traditionally been called *rales, rhonchi,* and *wheezes.* However, because of confusing and overlapping terminology and

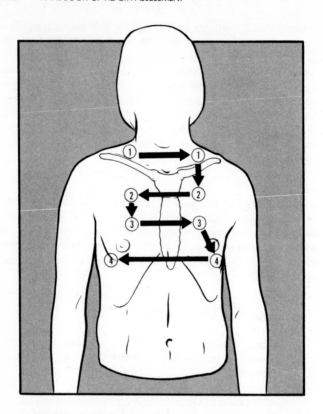

Figure 10–3. Pattern of chest percussion and auscultation.

lack of clinical consistency, the terms now recommended by the Joint Committee on Pulmonary Nomenclature describe adventitious breath sounds as "crackles" and "wheezes." Table 10–3 describes these sounds in more detail.

In describing abnormal or absent breath sounds, make careful note of the anatomical landmarks (rib number) and

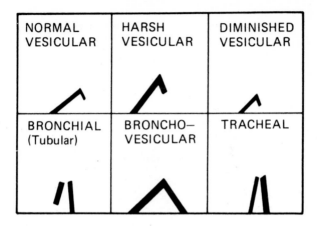

Figure 10–4. Normal breath sounds.

correlate this with the lobes of the lungs. Figure 10–6 shows the relationship of lung lobes to thoracic structures.

Voice Sounds
When abnormalities have been noted in either palpation for vocal fremitus, percussion for resonance, or auscultation for breath sounds, voice resonance should be assessed. Voice resonance is the transmission of sound through the chest wall as heard by the stethoscope. The most common voice sounds are listed in Table 10–4.

A decrease in voice resonance will occur in those conditions that cause a decrease in vocal fremitus, such as pneumothorax, atelectasis, and emphysema.

Recording

Normal
Thorax symmetrical with full equal expansion bilaterally. AP (anteroposterior) diameter greater than lateral, fremitus equal

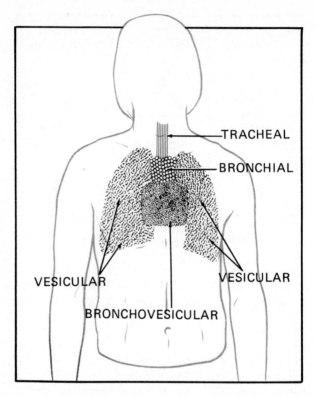

Figure 10–5. Areas of normal breath sounds.

bilaterally, resonant throughout lung fields. Vesicular breath sounds bilateral, no adventitious sounds.

Abnormal
Barrel chest with increased AP diameter, lung expansion equal bilaterally but diminished. Fremitus decreased bilaterally, lung fields hyperresonant except in area of left lower lobe in which

TABLE 10-3. ADVENTITIOUS SOUNDS (ABNORMAL SOUNDS)

Adventitious Sounds	Characteristics
CRACKLES	Defined as discrete, noncontinuous sounds. These may occur in inspiration or both inspiration and expiration.
Early inspiration crackles	Occur in conditions characterized by severe airway obstruction such as bronchitis, asthma, pulmonary emphysema. These early inspiratory crackles are usually few in number, low-pitched, vary in intensity, not cleared by coughing, audible at mouth as well as at bases.
Late inspiration crackles	Occur in conditions characterized by widespread pulmonary deflation such as pneumonia, pulmonary edema, and pulmonary fibrosis. These late inspiratory crackles are usually numerous, heard over chest wall, but not at the mouth, gravity dependent, making them change with position change.
	Late inspiratory crackles may also be present in the lung bases of patients on bedrest, in the elderly, or in some normal people and will clear with coughing. These are considered non-pathological, but support the need for coughing and deep breathing of immobile and postoperative patients.
Both inspiratory and expiratory crackles	Occur in conditions where both secretions and constricted airway passages interfere with air flow in both parts of the breathing cycle. Examples of this are in bronchiectasis and pulmonary edema. Crackles may also be accompanied by loud gurgling and bubbling sounds produced by secretions in the trachea and large bronchi.

(continued)

TABLE 10-3. ADVENTITIOUS SOUNDS (ABNORMAL SOUNDS) (Continued)

WHEEZES	Defined as continuous or musical sounds produced by the oscillation of narrowed bronchial walls as they open and close. The sound produced may be monophonic (single note) or polyphonic (several notes). Wheezes are typically expiratory, but may occur in both inspiration and expiration. Monophonic wheezes are associated with asthma and the single note produced may begin and end at different times during the breathing cycle. Polyphonic wheezes are associated with all types of obstructive lung disease and the several notes produced begin and end simultaneously during expiration.
FRICTION RUB	Sound described as rubbing or grating, due to inflamed pleural surfaces as in pleurisy, pneumonia, pulmonary infarction. The sound may resemble inspiratory crackles.

resonance is diminished. Breath sounds diminished with some crackling rales and expiratory wheezes in area just below scapulae on left posterior chest and at area of 6th rib on left anterior chest. Remainder of chest clear with distant but normal breath sounds; some prolongation of expiration.

The patient with these abnormal findings would be at high risk for the following nursing diagnosis:

Altered breathing pattern

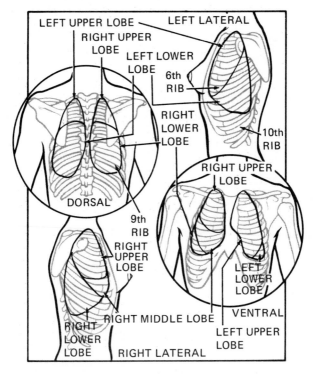

Figure 10–6. Anatomical relationship of lung lobes to thoracic cavity.

TABLE 10-4. ALTERED VOICE SOUNDS

Voice Sounds	Indications
Bronchophony	Patient says "99" and is normally indistinct on auscultation. May become more distinct with lung consolidation.
Whispered pectoriloquy	Patient whispers "1, 2, 3" which is normally inaudible on auscultation. Increased clarity and volume with lung consolidation.
Egophony	Patient says "e" which normally sounds like "e" on auscultation. With consolidation or pleural effusion the "e" sounds like "a" to the examiner.

Assessment of the Cardiovascular System

HEART

History Questions

Chest pain
   Description, location, onset, radiation, frequency
   Accompanying symptoms, relief
   Medications
Shortness of breath
   When you first noticed it
   When it bothers you most
   How far can you walk or exercise, number of stairs
   How relieved
   Medication
Difficulty breathing at night
   Number of pillows to sleep, recent change
Cough
   When you first noticed it
   Productive and description
Changes in heart rate or rhythm (palpitations)
Fatigue
   Activities you can no longer perform
   Daily rest required
Edema
   Recent weight changes
   Feet and hands edematous, in morning or evening

Extremities
  Coldness of extremities, tolerance of temperature
    changes
  Cyanosis, redness or other color changes of extremities
  Pain in extremities, description, onset, relieving factors
  Evidence of claudication, walking distance before pain
    begins, rest time needed to relieve pain, evidence of
    increasing severity
  Ulcers, difficulty healing
  Skin texture changes, loss of hair on extremities
  Change in shape and color of fingernails
  Varicose veins
    Location, onset
    Pain
    Use of support hose
  ECG
    Date and results
Problems with high blood pressure
  Headaches
  Dizziness or lightheaded on standing
Drugs
  Cardiac drugs
  Aspirin
Risk factors
  Smoking
  Stress
  Exercise
  Diet
    Cholesterol
    Salt

Examination

Vital Signs
Vital signs are usually done as soon as the patient is admitted.
If either the blood pressure or pulse is abnormal or if the chief
complaint warrants further investigation the blood pressure

and pulse should be repeated in a supine position, sitting and standing. If further abnormalities are found, the vital signs should be done in each arm. Differences between blood pressure reading in either arm or with position change (eg, supine to sitting) of 10 mm Hg or greater require further assessment; differences of less than 10 mm Hg are usually within normal variation (Figures 11–1 and 11–2).

Inspection

Inspect precordium and describe any pulsations, lifts, or rib retractions. Take particular note if apical pulsation is visible. Inspect internal jugular veins of neck, note pulsations and level of distention. No jugular distention should be seen with patient at 45° angle.

Examine nail beds for cyanosis and clubbing. Examples of nail clubbing have already been given in Table 3–4, p. 39. An easy way to quickly assess nail clubbing is to place the two

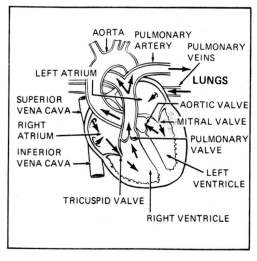

Figure 11–1. Internal anatomy of the heart.

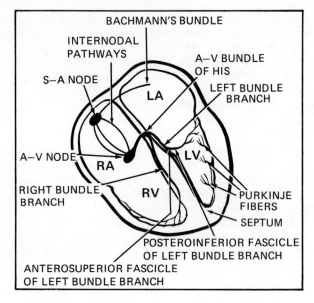

Figure 11–2. Conduction pathways of the heart. All labeled areas are part of conduction pathway beginning with SA node in the atrium and ending with the Purkinje fibers in the ventricles.

thumbs together with nailbeds facing. The loss of the nailbed angle becomes more apparent in this way. (See figure in Table 3–4).

Palpation

Palpate precordium (with cushioned part of hand at base of fingers (Figure 11–3). Proceed in orderly manner through the major areas of assessment for the heart:

Aortic area. 2nd intercostal space (ICS), right sternal border (RSB)

Pulmonic area. 2nd ICS, left sternal border (LSB)

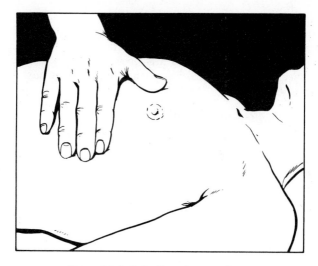

Figure 11–3. Palpation of precordium.

Tricuspid or right ventricular area. 4th or 5th ICS, left lower
  sternal border (LLSB)
Mitral or left ventricular area. 5th ICS—midclavicular line
  (MCL)

With palpation identify the point of maximum impulse
(PMI). This is generally at or near the mitral area but may be
displaced to the left with left ventricular hypertrophy. Record
the location of the apical impulse by interspace and relationship to midsternal line (MSL) or midclavicular line (MCL).
Identify any precordial thrills. These are caused by increased
blood turbulence and will herald the presence of a loud
murmur.

Percussion
Rarely used due to improvement in auscultatory equipment.

Auscultation

Auscultate at each of the five auscultatory sites in an organized manner with both the diaphragm and bell of the stethoscope (Figure 11–4). The diaphragm is designed to pick up high-pitched sounds, the bell, low-pitched sounds. The auscultatory sites are:

> *Aortic area* 2nd ICS, RSB
> *Pulmonic area* 2nd ICS, LSB

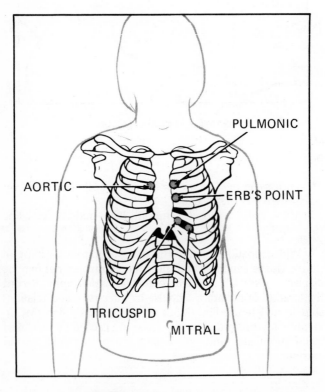

Figure 11–4. Auscultatory sites.

Erbs Point 3rd ICS, LSB
Tricuspid area 4th ICS, LLSB
Mitral (apical) area 5th ICS medial to MCL

First auscultate at each site with the diaphragm of the stethoscope and identify the first (S_1) and second (S_2) heart sounds. Recall that S_1 occurs just before the carotid pulse. Listening to the heart while feeling the carotid pulse may help in distinguishing between S_1 and S_2. Repeat the procedure, listening for extra sounds (S_3, S_4), murmurs, clicks, and friction rubs. Repeat the procedure of listening at each site, using the bell of the stethoscope.

Special Maneuvers

There are two special maneuvers to identify or rule out extra heart sounds or murmurs. (See Figure 11–5 for relationship of ECG complex to heart sounds.)

Left Lateral Decubitus Position *(use bell of stethoscope)*
    Patient is prone and asked to turn 45° to the left side; examiner may support patient's back to maintain this position. Both S_3, S_4 and mitral stenosis may be identified in this position.
Far Forward Front Upright *(use diaphragm of stethoscope)*
    Patient in a sitting position leans forward, exhales all air, and holds breath. Stethoscope at 2nd or 3rd intercostal space at left sternal border. Aortic insufficiency is often heard in this position.

Table 11–1 presents some defining characteristics of normal S_1 and S_2 and extra heart sounds including S_3, S_4, clicks, and snaps. Beginning practitioners should concentrate on identifying S_1 and S_2 and work on distinguishing extra heart sounds with increased practice time.

Murmurs

Heart murmurs are sounds caused by the turbulent flow of blood through the heart resulting in audible vibrations. Mur-

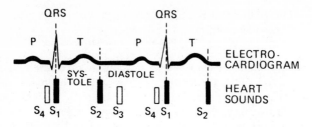

Figure 11–5. Relationship of ECG complex to heart sounds.

murs may be caused by (1) high flow through normal or abnormal valves; (2) forward flow through a constricted or irregular valve, or flow into a dilated area; or (3) backward flow through an incompetent valve, septal defect, or patent ductus arteriosus.

A heart murmur does not necessarily indicate organic pathology, but the examiner should take care to describe and record accurately the presence of all murmurs.

Murmurs should be described in the following manner:

    Location (anatomical)
    Quality
    Radiation
    Timing (in cardiac cycle)
    Loudness

Grading of murmurs is subjective, but the following scale is widely used and is helpful in rating the loudness of a murmur. Recording then is done as 3/6 to indicate grade 3 on a 6-point scale.

    Grade 1—very soft murmur
    Grade 2—easily heard murmur
    Grade 3—moderately loud murmur
    Grade 4—loud murmur may have accompanying thrill

Grade 5—loud murmur heard with stethoscope barely on chest

Grade 6—loud murmur heard with stethoscope off chest

The most common diastolic and systolic murmurs and a description of each are listed below.

SYSTOLIC MURMURS

The Innocent Systolic Murmur

"Innocent" systolic murmurs are murmurs produced by a normal cardiovascular system and are commonly heard in children and young adults. Innocent murmurs are always *systolic* and may occasionally be continuous. These murmurs are the ejection type, diamond shaped (crescendo, decrescendo), and usually the first part of systole.

Characteristics of Innocent Systolic Murmurs:

Innocent murmurs generally do not radiate

Innocent murmurs frequently disappear with inspiration or in the upright position

Innocent murmurs vary with the position of the patient

Innocent murmurs are usually softer than grade 3 out of 6

Heard best with bell of stethoscope

In the presence of any murmur, additional clues to cardiac pathology should be looked for carefully.

Mitral Regurgitation/Mitral Insufficiency

Common causes of mitral regurgitation:

Rheumatic heart disease

Papillary muscle dysfunction

Mitral valve prolapse

Ruptured chordae tendineae

Calcified mitral annulus

Left ventricular dilation (associated with left heart failure)

TABLE 11-1. NORMAL AND ABNORMAL HEART SOUNDS

Heart Sound	Characteristics
S_1 S_2	Occurs at beginning of ventricular contraction (systole) Associated with closure of mitral and tricuspid valves Usually heard best at apex or mitral area with *diaphragm* Nearly synchronous with carotid pulse
Split S_1 S_1 S_2	May be normally split at tricuspid area Abnormal splitting with right bundle branch block (RBBB) May be confused with ejection click or an S_4
S_2 S_1 S_2	Occurs with relaxation of ventricles (diastole) Associated with closure of aortic and pulmonic valves Usually heard best at aortic area with *diaphragm*
Split S_2 A_2 P_2 S_1 S_2 Normal Physiological Split of S_2	Due to delayed closure of pulmonic valve, heard on *inspiration.* Heard best in pulmonic area. If continues in expiration, will disappear in almost all normal subjects in semi-upright (40°) position In elderly individuals with split S_2 during expiration should signal possibility of disease

Fixed Split of S_2

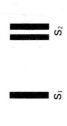

Components of S_2 (A,P) do not change with respirations. May be caused by:

RBBB
Left ventricular pacing
Pulmonic stenosis
Right ventricular failure (usually with pulmonary hypertension)
Atrial/septal defect
Idiopathic dilation of pulmonary artery
Mitral regurgitation
Ventricular-septal defect

Paradoxical Split of S_2

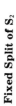

The usual sequence of valvular closure is aortic valve first followed by the pulmonic valve. In a paradoxical split the aortic valve closure is abnormally delayed causing the aortic valve closure to follow the pulmonic valve. This appears on expiration and disappears on inspiration. May be caused by:

LBBB
Aortic stenosis
Patent ductus arteriosis
Right ventricular pacing
Left ventricular failure or disease
Wolff-Parkinson-White syndrome, Type B (rare)

(continued)

TABLE 11-1. NORMAL AND ABNORMAL HEART SOUNDS (Continued)

Heart Sound	Characteristics
S_3 S_1 S_2 S_3	Termed a "Ventricular Gallop" Some describe the rhythm as sounding like "Ken-tuck-y" Occurs in diastole, after S_2 Heard best with bell of stethoscope at apex in left lateral decubitus position Normal in children, young adults, and females up to age 30 Almost always associated with heart disease in adults over 40 years old May be an early sign of congestive heart failure, decreased cardiac output May also occur due to increased velocity of blood flow in cases of severe anemia thyrotoxicosis, A-V shunts, and last trimester of pregnancy

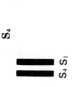

Termed an "Atrial Gallop" or "Atrial Diastolic Gallop" (both poor terms)

Some describe the rhythm as sounding like "Ten-nes-see"

Occurs in late diastole, before S_1

Heard best with bell at apex in left lateral decubitus position (lying on left side), may also be heard along left lower sternal border

Associated with decrease in ventricular compliance

May be caused by various conditions including:

Hypertensive cardiovascular disease

Myocardiopathy

Coronary artery disease, MI's

Aortic stenosis

Prolonged P-R intervals as in first-degree block

Pulmonary hypertension with cor pulmonale (right-sided S_4)

May also occur in severe anemias and hyperthyroidism

(continued)

TABLE 11-1. NORMAL AND ABNORMAL HEART SOUNDS (Continued)

Heart Sound	Characteristics
S_3 and S_4 S_1 $S_2 S_3 S_4 S_1$ $S_2 S_3 S_4$	Termed "Summation Gallop" When both extra sounds are present and heart rate is rapid, these two sounds fuse to produce a mid-diastolic sound, which is the summation (sum of S_3 and S_4) Gallop Rhythm May be confused with diastolic murmur due to the "rumble" quality Heard best with bell at apex in left lateral decubitus position
Aortic Ejection Sounds S_1 E_J S_2	Heard best with diaphragm at lower apex Need to differentiate this sound from S_4; this sound will not vary with change in patient position Commonly heard with: Aortic valvular stenosis (usually congenital type) Aortic insufficiency Coarctation of the aorta
Pulmonic Ejection Sounds S_1 E_J S_2	Heard best with diaphragm along upper LSB; loudest during expiration Simulates a split S_1 but varies with respirations Heard best at pulmonic area so this sound r/o split S_1 Heard with: Pulmonary stenosis Pulmonary hypertension Dilation of pulmonary artery

Systolic Clicks

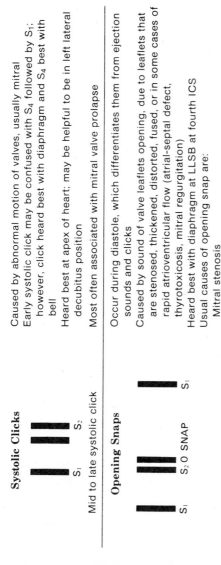

Caused by abnormal motion of valves, usually mitral

Early systolic click may be confused with S_4 followed by S_1; however, click heard best with diaphragm and S_4 best with bell

Heard best at apex of heart; may be helpful to be in left lateral decubitus position

Most often associated with mitral valve prolapse

S_1 S_2

Mid to late systolic click

Opening Snaps

Occur during diastole, which differentiates them from ejection sounds and clicks

Caused by sound of valve leaflets opening, due to leaflets that are stenosed, thickened, distorted, fused, or in some cases of rapid atrioventricular flow (atrial-septal defect, thyrotoxicosis, mitral regurgitation)

Heard best with diaphragm at LLSB at fourth ICS

Usual causes of opening snap are:

Mitral stenosis

Tricuspid stenosis

S_1 S_2 O SNAP

S_1

Opening snaps may be difficult to distinguish from a split S_2 and even an S_3

If an extra sound is heard in early systole, it is called an "ejection sound or ejection click" because it coincides with the onset of ventricular systolic ejection. However, a sound heard in mid- or late systole is termed a "systolic click" since it occurs after the onset of ejection. The terms are confusing and often interchanged.

Description

> Location: apex, heard best with diaphragm, may increase
>   after exercise
> Quality: swoosh, blowing diaphragm
> Radiation: axilla (except elderly with sclerosis)
> Timing: Systolic, often pansystolic, steady intensity

(See Figure 11–6.)

Aortic Stenosis

Common causes of aortic stenosis:

> Rheumatic fever
> Congenital aortic valve disease

Description:

> Location: Aortic site and LSB, sometimes apex
>   Heard best in front forward position with diaphragm
> Quality: Harsh (diaphragm)
> Radiation: Carotid, neck clavicle
> Timing: Systolic, diamond-shaped, ends before S_2

(See Figure 11–7.)

Figure 11–6. Mitral regurgitation.

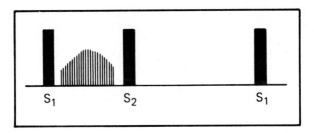

Figure 11–7. Aortic stenosis.

Less Common Systolic Murmurs Include:

Tricuspid insufficiency (regurgitation)
Pulmonic stenosis
Ventricular septal defect

DIASTOLIC MURMURS

Mitral Stenosis
Causes of mitral stenosis are:

Calcification of the valve leaflet or dense scarring
Subvalvular fusion or commissural fusion

The causes of these valvular changes are usually due to:

Rheumatic heart disease
Congenital valvular disease

Description:

Location: Apex, may need patient in left lateral decubitus
    position *(use bell of stethoscope)*
Quality: Rumble, low pitched
Radiation: None

Timing: Early to mid-diastole, an opening snap may
accompany the murmur; the opening snap occurs after
S_2 and before S_3

(See Figure 11–8.)

Aortic Insufficiency (Regurgitation)
Common causes of aortic insufficiency:

Rheumatic heart disease
Aortic root dissection
Hypertension
Arteriosclerosis
Congenital aortic valvular disease
Ascending aortic aneurysm (suspect this if new develop-
ment and patient has diastolic hypertension)
Sinus of Valsalva aneurysm
Marfan's syndrome
Endocarditis
Tertiary syphillis

Description

Location: LLSB, second right intercostal space, use diaphragm
Quality: Wind in trees, blowing

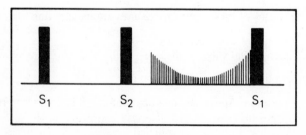

Figure 11–8. Mitral stenosis.

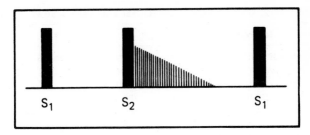

Figure 11–9. Aortic insufficiency (regurgitation).

Radiation: Neck
Timing: After S_2 in early diastole. May not hear the S_2.
  May need to have patient sit up, lean forward, blow out
  air.

(See Figure 11–9.)

PERIPHERAL VASCULAR

Examination

Inspection and Palpation

Upper Extremities. Inspect both arms, noting color, skin temperature, texture of skin, hair distribution or lack of hair, venous patterns, and edema. Palpate radial and brachial arteries, noting rate and rhythm, comparing volume and patency between sides (Figure 11–10).

Perform Allen test to check patency of radial and ulnar arteries if occlusion is suspected. This test is of particular importance in patients requiring frequent arterial punctures for blood gas analysis. Table 11–2 lists four special maneuvers to test the vascular system.

TABLE 11-2. SPECIAL MANEUVERS TO TEST VASCULAR SYSTEM

Test Maneuver	Results
Allen test: With hand raised, have patient clench fist tightly, occlude radial artery with examiner's thumb. Then have patient open the hand in a relaxed position. Repeat test and occlude ulnar artery to determine patency of radial artery.	The color of the palms should promptly return to a normal color. Persistence of pallor indicates occlusion of the ulnar artery (artery not being compressed by examiner).

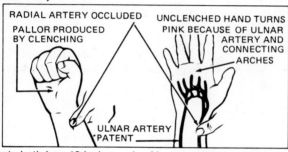

RADIAL ARTERY OCCLUDED
PALLOR PRODUCED BY CLENCHING

UNCLENCHED HAND TURNS PINK BECAUSE OF ULNAR ARTERY AND CONNECTING ARCHES

ULNAR ARTERY PATENT

Elevate both legs 12 inches and move feet up and down at ankles 30–60 seconds.	Maneuver removes venous blood, increased or unusual pallor of extremities indicates poor arterial blood supply to legs, arterial insufficiency.
Following above maneuver have patient sit up and dangle legs.	Color should return in 10 seconds, veins in feet and ankles should fill in 15 seconds. Delay of these indicate poor arterial response.
Homan's sign: Dorsiflex foot with leg flat on bed.	Presence of calf pain with this maneuver suggests phlebitis.
Squeeze large calf muscles against tibia.	Tenderness, increased firmness, or edema. Suggests deep phlebitis.

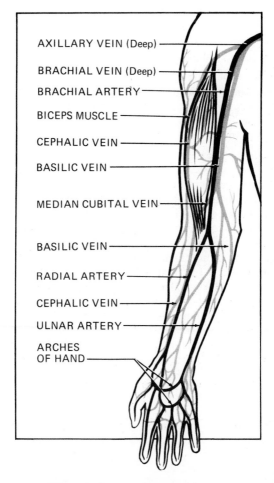

Figure 11–10. Major arteries of the arm.

Lower Extremities. Inspect legs and feet noting color, skin temperature, texture of skin, hair distribution or lack of hair, venous patterns and edema. Palpate femoral, popliteal, posterior tibial, and dorsalis pedis pulses. Note volume, patency, and equality of sides (Figure 11–11).

Pulses are most frequently described as normal, diminished, or absent. However, when a rating scale is used it usually includes 0 to 4 with the following rating:

0 = absent
1 = barely palpable or markedly impaired
2 = diminished or moderately impaired
3 = slightly impaired
4 = normal

Peripheral vascular disorders can be caused by disorders of the lymphatic, venous, and arterial systems. Common findings in peripheral vascular disease include pain, paresthesia, edema, skin changes, and ulcerations.

Whenever edema is encountered in a physical examination the extent of the edema should be noted along with any accompanying symptoms (eg, redness, tenderness). Also, there is usually an attempt to describe the severity of the edema by grading it from a 1+ (minimal) to 4+ (severe pitting edema). This grading, however, lacks consistency between individuals but can provide a benchmark for judging improvement.

Table 11–3 summarizes the most common characteristics of peripheral vascular disease affecting the arterial and venous systems. It is not uncommon for patients to exhibit symptoms of both arterial and venous insufficiency.

Recording Cardiovascular

Normal

No lifts or heaves, apical impulse palpable at 5th ICS, MCL; no thrills; rate 72, regular; $S_1 > S_2$ at apex, no extra sounds, murmurs or rubs.

Abnormal

Carotid pulse visible, slight jugular venous distension at 45°; heave at apex, apical impulse 6th ICS anterior axillary line, no

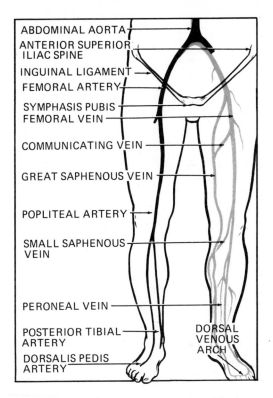

Figure 11–11. Major veins and arteries of the leg.

thrills; rate 120, regular; $S_1 > S_2$, grade 2/6 blowing; pansystolic murmur at 5th ICS, MCL, radiates to left axilla.

The patient with these abnormal findings would be at high risk for the following nursing diagnoses:

Decreased cardiac output
Potential alteration in cardiopulmonary tissue perfusion
Anxiety
Potential activity intolerance

TABLE 11-3. COMPARISONS OF CHRONIC ARTERIAL INSUFFICIENCY AND CHRONIC VENOUS INSUFFICIENCY

Symptoms Elicited From Health History	Chronic Arterial Insufficiency	Chronic Venous Insufficiency
Response to Exercise	Easy fatigability. Intermittent claudication (pain with exercise, relieved with rest; in the arms may be confused with pain of angina pectoris)	Aching pain in calf or areas of venous stasis, particularly after standing for some time
Coldness of Extremities	May feel cold due to lack of adequate blood supply	May feel cold due to associated vasospasms and pooled venous blood that loses heat
Paresthesia (numbness, tingling in extremities)	Often described in a "stocking-glove" distribution and must be differentiated from neurological disorders	May report some numbness or tingling, but not as common as in arterial insufficiency

Pulses	Diminished or absent (absence of femoral pulse plus one peripheral pulse is sufficient criteria for diagnosis of arterial insufficiency)	Present (may be difficult to assess if edema is profound)
Color of Extremities	Pallor of extremity, especially with elevation. With dependency extremity may be cyanotic due to poor arterial circulation or appear dusky red (cyanotic rubor)	Normal or cyanotic with dependency due to pooled venous blood
Skin	Skin atrophy and loss of hair follicles, oil and sweat glands in affected skin. This results in thin, shiny looking skin, sparse hair or loss of hair, no perspiration, and dry, cracked skin. Nail beds develop longitudinal ridges, become thickened and curve over the tip of the finger or toe (ramshead nails)	Brown mottling or pigmentation around ankles. This is caused by tiny purpuric lesions in the ankle that resolve and leave iron pigments in the skin causing a brownish color. Itching may accompany these skin changes
Ulcers	May develop at pressure points on feet (often the toes) or lateral of surface of leg. In patients with Raynaud's syndrome, ulceration may occur at the side of the finger near the base of the nail	Above the malleolus, most often the inner ankle (medial malleolus)

(continued)

TABLE 11-3. COMPARISONS OF CHRONIC ARTERIAL INSUFFICIENCY AND CHRONIC VENOUS INSUFFICIENCY (Continued)

Symptoms Elicited From Health History	Chronic Arterial Insufficiency	Chronic Venous Insufficiency
Skin Temperature (Very difficult to evaluate accurately in physical exam as room temperature has large effect on skin temperature.)	Cool	Normal
Gangrene	May occur as a result of prolonged tissue ischemia, usually from trombolic occlusion of distal branches of arteries	Generally not associated with gangrene. However, venous obstruction may cause secondary superficial arterial lesions resulting in gangrene

Recording Peripheral Vascular

Normal
Extremities warm to touch with normal hair distribution. No venous dilation. Temporal, carotid, radial, brachial, femoral, popliteal, posterior tibial, and dorsalis pedis pulses equal and of good quality. No carotid or femoral bruits present.

Abnormal
Legs cool to the touch, pale, and faintly mottled. Hair diminished from mid-calf to ankles bilaterally. Toes without hairs, toenails thick with horizontal ridges. Femoral pulses present and equal. Dorsalis pedis and popliteal pulses not palpable. No femoral bruits present.

The patient with abnormal findings would be at high risk for the following nursing diagnosis:

Altered peripheral tissue perfusion

12 | Assessment of the Abdomen

History Questions

Pain in abdomen
  Location, quality, quantity, timing, setting, aggravating, alleviating, and associated factors
Change in appetite
  Weight loss or gain
Chewing and swallowing problems
Heartburn
  Frequency
  Antacids
Nausea, vomiting, regurgitation
Rectal bleeding
  Frequency
  Color: Bright red or tarry stools
Elimination
  Constipation
  Diarrhea
  Change in shape of stool
  Roughage
  Cathartics, enemas
  Change in bowel habits
Hemorrhoids
  Pain
  Itching
  Bleeding

Voiding difficulty
   Pain or burning
   Force in stream
   Nocturia
Previous surgery
   Residual problems

(Figure 12–1 illustrates anatomy of abdominal cavity.)

Pain is often experienced by the patient with abdominal problems. The schematic of segments of the spinal cord that innervate the visceral organs and conduct pain sensations is presented in Figure 12–2.

Examination

Inspection

Inspect skin for scars, rashes, lesions, turgor, striae, venous structure, color, petechiae.

Inspect architecture (or contour) and describe:
Protuberant: obese, rounded, distended
Scaphoid: concave, navicular
Symmetry: Masses and deformity will distort; having the supine patient lift head off bed will display ventral hernia.

Inspect umbilicus for protrusion, retraction, discoloration (bluish color may indicate blood in peritoneal cavity), drainage, fistula.

Inspect for pulsations and peristaltic waves.

Auscultation

This technique is performed before percussion and palpation in order to negate alteration of bowel sounds.

Auscultate for evidence of bowel sounds. Use the diaphragm of the stethoscope lightly and listen in all four quadrants. Before reporting the absence of bowel sounds, listen carefully in all quadrants for five minutes.

Right Upper Quadrant	Left Upper Quadrant
Right lobe of liver	Left lobe of liver
Gallbladder	Spleen
Pylorus	Stomach
Duodenum	Left kidney
Head of the pancreas	Body and tail of pancreas
Upper part of right kidney	Splenic flexure of colon
Hepatic flexure of colon	

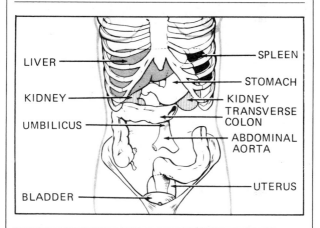

Right Lower Quadrant	Left Lower Quadrant
Lower portion of right kidney	Sigmoid colon
Cecum	Left fallopian tube
Appendix	Left ovary
Ascending colon	Left ureter
Right fallopian tube	Midline
Right ovary	Uterus
Right ureter	Urinary bladder

Figure 12–1. Anatomy of abdominal cavity.

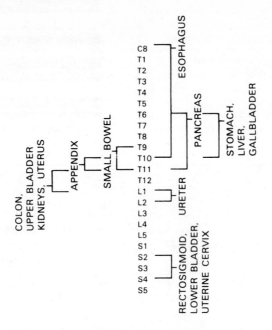

Figure 12–2. Segments of the spinal cord that innervate visceral organs and conduct pain sensations. (*From Capell P.T. and Case, D.C. Ambulatory Care Manual for Nurse Practitioners. J.B. Lippincott Co., Philadelphia, 1976, with permission.*)

Evaluate pitch and intensity of sounds. Listen for abnormal sounds:

Increased frequency and intensity of bowel sounds (borborygmi) in enteritis or small bowel obstruction;
Loud and continuous sounds in bacterial and viral enteritis;
Peristaltic rushes and metallic tinkling sounds alternating with periods of silence in bowel obstruction;

Rough grating sounds of peritoneal friction rub from an inflamed visceral peritoneum.

Auscultate for bruits, which are heard most often in cardiac systole. Abdominal bruits are typically soft sounds and can easily be missed. Listen:

Between the xiphoid process and the umbilicus for bruits due to aneurysm of the abdominal aorta;

Over the flank areas or costovertebral angles for renal artery stenosis;

Over the liver for the continuous venous hum of cirrhosis.

Percussion

Percuss lightly in all four quadrants to assess general proportion and distribution of tympany and dullness.

Percuss the liver:

In the right mid-clavicular line (MCL), starting below the umbilicus (and percussing upward at MCL toward the liver to determine lower border liver dullness);

In the right mid-clavicular line from lung resonance down toward liver dullness. Measure in centimeters the vertical height of liver dullness;

Percussion may outline the liver boundaries in the right mid-sternal area also;

It should be noted that liver heights are generally greater in men than women and in the tall, as opposed to the short, individual. Normal liver heights at the mid-clavicular line are 6–12 cm and 4–8 at the mid-sternal line (Figure 12–3).

Percuss over the left lower anterior rib cage to identify the tympany of the gastric air bubble.

Percuss for tympany in the lowest interspace in the left anterior axillary line. Ask the patient to take a deep breath; if continued percussion reveals the same tympany note, the spleen is probably normal in size.

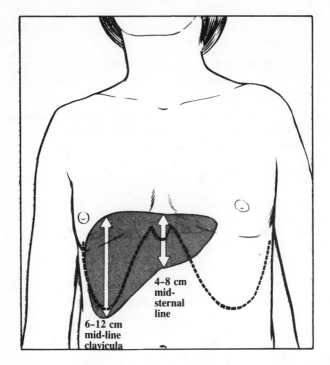

Figure 12–3. Normal liver heights.

Palpation
Palpate lightly initially in all four quadrants away from pain to identify abdominal tenderness and superficial masses. Then palpate deeply in all quadrants to delineate abdominal organs and masses.

Palpate for *masses* and note location, size, shape, consistency, tenderness, pulsations, mobility.

Palpate for *rebound tenderness* (by firmly and slowly pressing in and quickly withdrawing fingers).

Palpation of Liver

Place fingertips below the lower border of liver dullness, pointing toward right costal margin and have the patient take a deep breath. Feel the liver edge as it descends on inspiration (Figure 12–4).

Palpation of Spleen

Palpate in the lower left rib cage for the spleen by placing the patient on the right side with legs bent for gravity to bring spleen into palpable location. *The spleen must be enlarged to three times its normal size to be palpable.*

Palpate for aortic pulsations in the upper abdomen slightly left to the mid-line.

Palpation of Kidney

Palpate the left kidney by placing the left hand at the patient's left posterior costal angle and the right hand at the left anterior costal margin. Instruct the patient to take a deep breath and exhale completely. As the patient exhales, elevate the patient's left flank with the left hand and palpate deeply with the right hand. Rarely will the kidney be palpable. Repeat the same procedure to examine the right kidney.

Recording

Normal

Flat with no visible pulsations, lesions or hernias; bowel sounds present and active in all four quadrants; no bruits or CVA tenderness. Liver edge at costal margin is smooth and non-tender; liver height 9 cm at MCL. Abdominal tympany in left upper quadrant. No tenderness or palpable masses. Spleen and kidneys not palpated.

Abnormal

Flat with no visible lesions or pulsations. Bowel sounds present in all four quadrants. Localized tenderness and muscular rigidity present in right lower quadrant extending to the

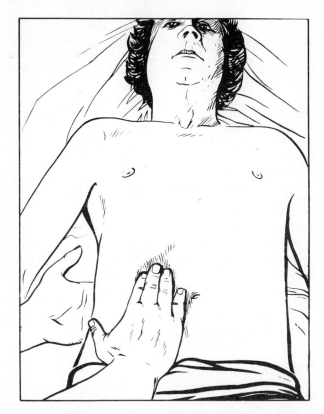

Figure 12–4. Technique for liver palpation.

right flank. Severe pain in right lower quadrant when left quadrant palpated; referred rebound tenderness also present. Psoas sign positive. Liver height 8 cm at MCL. Spleen and kidneys not palpable.

The patient with these abnormal findings would be at high risk for the following diagnoses:

Pain
Potential for infection

13 | Assessment of the Musculoskeletal System

History Questions

Muscle size and strength
    Change in size of arms and/or legs
    Changes in strength, activities of daily living (ADL)
    Muscle cramping, at rest, walking or with exercise
Joint mobility
    Morning stiffness, related to weight bearing or particular activities
    Deformities, discoloration
    Stiffness, redness, swelling
    Arthritis, gout
Change in sensation
    Vibratory, temperature, light touch
Bones
    Deformities
    History of fractures, orthopedic surgery
Pain
    Backache, muscle soreness, joints
    At rest or with exercise

Skeletal pain is often difficult to differentiate from visceral pain, making the assessment of the patient with musculoskeletal problems difficult to achieve. Table 13–1 will assist the examiner in differentiating between skeletal and visceral pain.

Once the diagnosis of skeletal pain is established, further investigation is necessary to determine if the pain is related or

TABLE 13-1. CHARACTERISTICS OF SKELETAL PAIN AND VISCERAL PAIN

Skeletal	Visceral
1. Local tenderness to touch	1. Associated cardiorespiratory or abdominal symptoms, eg, wheezing, dyspnea, nausea, vomiting
2. Pain on simple motion, often reduced by decreased movement	2. Pain may be present or worsened without movement
3. Normal or stable vital signs	3. Abnormal or unstable vital signs. May elicit autonomic reflexes, eg, vagal slowing of heart rate
4. Pattern not characteristic of visceral pain	4. May have a characteristic pattern, eg, anginal, pleuritic
5. May follow trauma, exercise, emotional disturbance	5. May have antecedent history suggesting specific visceral origin

From: Capell, P.T. and Case, D.C. *Ambulatory Care Manual for Nurse Practitioners.* J.B. Lippincott Co., Philadelphia, 1976, with permission.

unrelated to joints. Figure 13–1 will assist the examiner with this investigation.

Examination

Inspection and Palpation
General approach.

> Note active and passive ROM
>> Note any swelling, deformity
>> Listen for crepitation or grating as joint moves
>> Note muscle strength, atrophy, hypertrophy
>> Note condition of surrounding tissues, skin changes, subcutaneous nodules
>> Note symmetry.

Back and Vertebral Column With Patient Standing
Figure 13–2 illustrates lateral view of vertebral column.

> Note *normal curves:* Cervical concavity, thoracic convexity, lumbar concavity
> Palpate for tenderness around the spinous processes and paravertebral muscles, note any muscle spasms
> Standing behind patient note:
>> Any sacral edema
>> Lateral curve (scoliosis), if present
>> Differences in height of shoulders and iliac crests
> With patient touching toes note:
>> Symmetry
>> Flattening of lumbar curve
>> ROM
> While stabilizing patient's pelvis, note ability to bend sideways, bend backwards, twist shoulders.
> Head and upper extremities with patient sitting
>> Head and neck
>> Inspect neck for abnormalities and deformities
>> Palpate temporomandibular joint; assess tenderness around spinous processes and paravertebral muscles

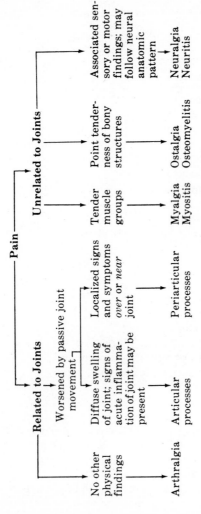

Figure 13–1. Approach to musculoskeletal pain. *(From Capell, P.T. and Case, D.C. Ambulatory Care Manual for Nurse Practitioners. J.B. Lippincott Co., Philadelphia, 1976, with permission.)*

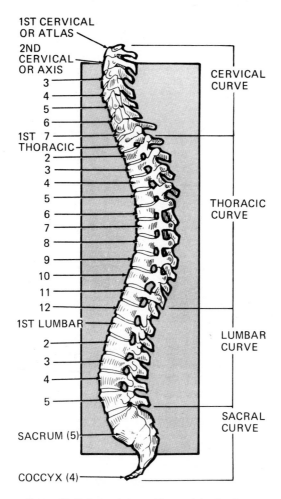

Figure 13–2. Lateral view of the vertebral column.

Assess ROM: Flexion, extension, rotation, lateral bending

Hands and Wrists

Inspect for swelling, redness, nodules, deformities

Palpate each joint

Assess ROM: Extend and spread fingers; make fist with thumbs across fingers; flex, extend, abduct and adduct wrists

Elbows

Inspect around olecranon, and humeral epicondyles

Palpate around olecranon, and humeral epicondyles

Assess ROM: Flex, extend, pronate, supinate

Shoulders

Inspect anteriorly and posteriorly

Palpate sternoclavicular joint, acromioclavicular joint, entire shoulder

Assess ROM: Flexion, extension, abduction, adduction, internal rotation, external rotation

Figure 13–3 illustrates the structure of a synovial joint.

Lower Extremities With Patient Lying Down

Feet and Ankles

Inspect ankle joint, Achilles' tendon, remaining joints

Asess ROM: dorsiflexion, plantar flexion, inversion, eversion, flexion and extension of toes

Knees

Inspect for alignment, status of quadriceps, loss of normal hollows around the patella

Palpate suprapatellar pouch

Assess ROM: Flexion and extension

Hips and Pelvis

Inspect for symmetry

Assess ROM: With knees flexed—flexion, extension, internal, external rotation; with knees extended—flexion, extension, hyperextension, abduction, adduction. *Note:* These maneuvers should be done with

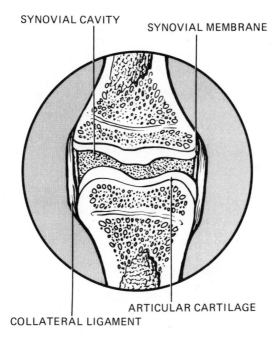

SYNOVIAL CAVITY   SYNOVIAL MEMBRANE

ARTICULAR CARTILAGE

COLLATERAL LIGAMENT

Figure 13–3. The basic structure of a synovial joint.

extreme caution on patients who have had recent hip replacements.

Figure 13–4 illustrates six basic types of synovial joints.

Deep Tendon Reflexes

General Principles
Assist patient to relax
Position limb so muscle is mildly stretched
Strike tendon briskly, holding hammer loosely yet with
control

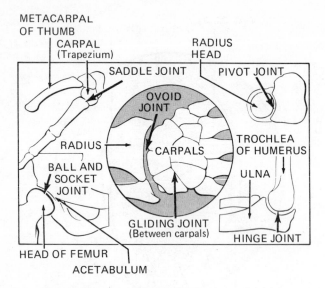

Figure 13–4. The six basic types of synovial joints, illustrated by joints of the body.

Compare responses in symmetrical manner, side to side
Use following symbols to indicate response:
+ + + + hyperactive
+ + + brisker than normal
+ + normal
+ hypoactive
0 absent
Try *reinforcement techniques* if reflex is difficult to elicit:
Ask patient to change position;
Ask patient to hook fingers together and, on command, pull them in opposite directions while examiner attempts to elicit reflexes of *lower extremities;*
Ask patient to clench one fist tightly while examiner attempts to elicit reflexes in *opposite arm.*

Note: See neurological examination for complete tendon reflex assessment, pp. 199–200.

Recording

Normal
Posture erect with normal lumbar lordosis; no palpable or visible muscle tightness or spasm. Full ROM of hands, wrists, elbows, shoulders, spine, hips, knees, and ankles. Normal gait with equal stride. Can walk on heel and toe. Straight leg raising painless to limits of hamstring tightness. Reflexes equal. No motor or sensory deficit. Sciatic nerves not tender on deep palpation. No pain or palpation over bony processes.

Abnormal
Radicular pain with numbness and weakness in right leg. Loss of lordosis in erect and prone positions. Raising uninvolved leg produces pain in involved leg. Sciatic nerve tender to deep palpation. Hyperesthesia, motor weakness, and diminution of DTRs present in right leg. Full ROM in joints of upper extremities.

The patient with these abnormal findings would be at high risk for the following nursing diagnoses:

Pain
Impaired physical mobility
Potential activity intolerance

14 | Assessment of Female Genitalia and Rectum

History Questions

Menses
  Age of menarche
  Cycle description
    Frequency, duration, irregularity, amount of flow
  Dysmenorrhea, primary or secondary
  Spotting between periods
  Date of last menstrual period
Menopause
  Age of last menstrual period
  Climacteric symptoms
    Change or cessation of periods, flushing, palpitations
    Sweats, vaginal dryness
Pregnancies
  Mode of delivery
  Anesthesia
  Problems, complications
  Birth weight of children, and gestational ages
  Problem getting pregnant
  Activity
  Type of contraception
Vaginal discharge
  Description, treatment, outcome
Sexually transmitted diseases
  Gonorrhea, syphilis, herpes, scabies; course of illness,

specific treatment, outcome
Painful sores or blisters on external genitals, inner thigh,
buttocks, or groin
Sexual functioning
Activity, changes, problems
Bleeding or pain during intercourse *(dyspareunia)*
Satisfactory sexual adjustment
Number of sexual partners
Any exposure to partners with high risk for HIV infec-
tion
General
Douching practices
Last Pap test and result
Medications

Figure 14–1 illustrates the exterior anatomy of female
genitalia.

Facts on Normal Menstrual Patterns

Menstruation usually begins between the ages of 9 and 16.
Factors that affect age of *menarche* (onset of menstrual
pattern):
Family history (menarche of mother, sisters)
Race (white girls generally have earlier menarche)
Nutritional status, especially level of body fat (low body
fat may delay menarche)
Usual range of days between menses is 24 to 32.
Many girls do not have a regular pattern for a year or
more after they begin menstruating.
High levels of exercise can cause skipped period, and
even complete loss of menses *(amenorrhea)*.
Extreme weight loss can also cause loss of menstrual
periods.
Menstrual flow is usually 3 to 7 days.
Scanty flow or infrequent menstrual flow is *oligomenor-
rhea*.
Mild discomfort with menses is not unusual; cramping

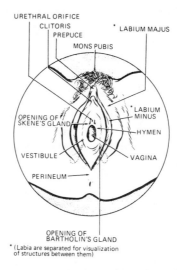

URETHRAL ORIFICE
CLITORIS
PREPUCE
MONS PUBIS
* LABIUM MAJUS
* LABIUM MINUS
HYMEN
OPENING OF SKENE'S GLAND
VAGINA
VESTIBULE
PERINEUM
OPENING OF BARTHOLIN'S GLAND
* (Labia are separated for visualization of structures between them)

Figure 14-1. Exterior anatomy of female genitalia.

or severe pain when menstruating is called *dysmenorrhea.*

Menopause is the cessation of menstrual periods and occurs around 45 to 52 years of age. Changes in menstrual flow (either heavier or scant) and skipped periods often accompany the onset of menopause. Other symptoms associated with menopause are hot flashes, and flushing and sweating with these hot flashes.

Examination
This part of the physical examination should be done near the completion of the examination so that the patient has had time to relax and establish some rapport with the examiner. The

patient should have an empty bladder for the examination. Explain each step in the examination as you perform it. This is particularly important with the insertion of the speculum, and the bimanual and rectovaginal exams.

External Genitalia

Inspection and Palpation
Note hair distribution, identify anatomical landmarks of external genitalia, looking for lacerations, lesions, edema, hematomas, masses, and discharge.

With gloved hand separate the labia majora. Insert finger into vagina to milk urethra for discharge from Skene's glands; palpate area of Bartholin's glands for pain or discharge (Figure 14–2).

Move two fingers inside the vagina and separate opening. Ask patient to bear down and observe for bulging of the anterior (cystocele) or posterior (rectocele) wall of the vagina or incontinence of urine.

Internal Genitalia

Inspection
Speculum exam. A speculum of the proper size should be lubricated and warmed by running warm water over it (commonly used jelly lubricants can interfere with results of Pap test or other cytological studies).

Insert speculum using following steps:

1. Place two fingers (R hand) just inside or at introitus of vagina, gently pressing down (Figure 14–3).
2. Introduce closed speculum (other hand) past fingers at 45° angle down and posteriorly holding blades obliquely (Figure 14–4).
3. Advance speculum by putting pressure on posterior vaginal wall.
4. After speculum has entered vagina, remove fingers and rotate blades to horizontal position (Figure 14–5).

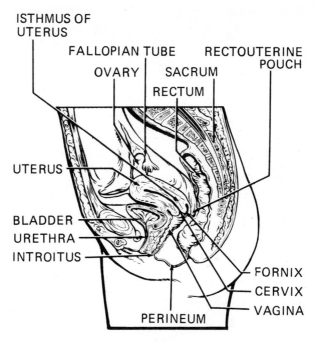

Figure 14–2. Interior anatomy of female genitalia.

5. Open the blades after full insertion and maneuver until cervix is in full view (Figure 14–6).
6. Adjust speculum to remain in open position (Figure 14–7).

Inspect *vagina* for color, discharge, lesions (Table 14–1 lists common vaginal discharges).

Inspect *cervix* for description of os, color, erosions, lacerations, and discharge.

Perform *Papanicolaou Test* for cervical cytology if part of examination (Figure 14–8).

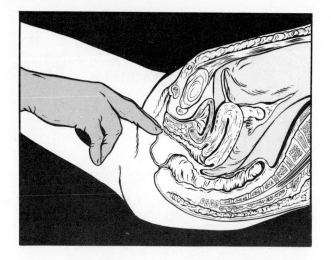

Figure 14–3. Fingers at introitus of vagina.

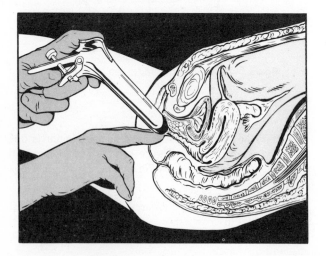

Figure 14–4. Insertion of speculum.

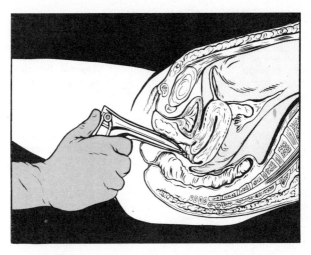

Figure 14–5. Rotation of speculum blades to horizontal position.

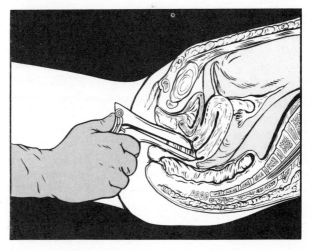

Figure 14–6. Opening of speculum blades.

TABLE 14-1. COMMON VAGINAL DISCHARGES

Characteristics of Discharge	Patient Symptoms	Probable Causes
Clear discharge changing to thick, white viscous discharge	None	Normal; first two weeks after menses discharge is clear changing to thicker white after ovulation.
Thick white curdlike or cheesy appearing discharge, adheres to vaginal wall, usually little odor	Itching, inflamed vulva	Monilia (Candida); treated with vaginal suppositories. This is a yeast infection and symptomatic relief enhanced with baking soda douches.
Profuse yellow or greenish-gray, often frothy and foul-smelling discharge, vaginal wall and cervix may have red granular (strawberry spots) or petechiae spots	Profuse, foul discharge, itching, inflamed vulva.	Trichomonas vaginalis; treated with oral medication; consider treating patient's sexual partner to prevent "ping-pong" effect of reinfection.
Yellow to greenish discharge often with inflamed urethra and Bartholin's glands. Cervix may be inflamed with yellowish discharge from os	Change in vaginal discharge and painful urination.	Gonorrhea; treated routinely with penicillin unless patient is allergic. Sexual partner(s) must be treated also. Routine cultures are important when

TABLE 14-1. COMMON VAGINAL DISCHARGES (Continued)

Characteristics of Discharge	Patient Symptoms	Probable Causes
		gonorrhea is suspected, even in the absence of symptoms, as most females are asymptomatic until PID (pelvic inflammatory disease) occurs.
Thin, whitish, blood-tinged discharge. No external inflammation	Vaginal dryness, painful intercourse, often with bleeding	Atrophic (senile) vaginitis; treat with vaginal cream or low-level hormones.
Increased amounts of white viscous discharge	Rarely itching and burning, discharge often has "fishy" odor	Gardenella vaginalis (non-specific vaginitis) This is a sexually transmitted anaerobic organism. Both partners should be treated with oral or topical medication.
White, viscous cervical discharge	Often asymptomatic	Chlamydia Trachomatis (non-gonococcal vaginitis); oral antibiotics for both partners

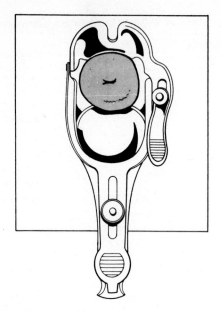

Figure 14–7. Speculum in open position to view cervix.

1. *Cervical os.* Insert cotton-tipped applicator into opening of cervix. Roll between fingers to pick up discharge. Smear gently onto glass slide. Use proper fixation agent immediately.
2. *Cervical scrape.* With special spatula, place long end into cervical os and rotate spatula around entire cervical opening in a scraping manner. Smear spatula onto glass slide. Use proper fixation agent immediately.
3. *Vaginal pool.* Insert cotton-tipped applicator into poste-

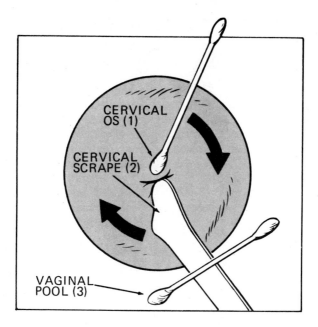

Figure 14–8. Papanicolaou test.

rior fornix where the vaginal pool is located below the cervix. Smear gently onto glass slide. Use proper fixation agent immediately.

Note: The inside of the cervix is lined with columnar epithelium; the outside of the cervix is covered with squamous epithelium. Most cancers begin at the squamo-columnar junction near the cervical os. Proper scraping of cells at this area is vital to proper cytology tests (Figure 14–9).

If cervix has been surgically removed, perform a scrape from the vaginal cuff and obtain a specimen from the vaginal pool.

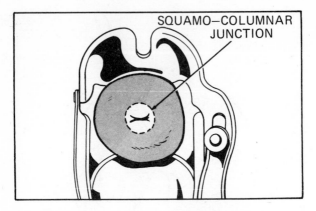

Figure 14–9. Squamo-columnar junction of cervix.

Palpation

Bimanual exam. The examiner is in a standing position and inserts gloved and lubricated index and middle fingers with pressure on posterior surface. Turn finger pads to face anterior wall. Palpate vaginal wall. Note firmness, tenderness, masses, bulging of wall.

Palpate *cervix*. Note contour, tenderness, mobility, masses or nodules (Figure 14–10).

Palpate *uterus* by pressing downward on abdominal wall with outside hand while pushing upward on either side of cervix with two fingers in vagina. Note size, shape, position, consistency, mobility, and tenderness (Figure 14–11).

Palpate *ovaries* by pressing downward with hand on abdomen and upward with fingers in vagina at each side of uterus. This should be a stroking motion with the fingers of both hands pushing together as the hands are moved downward. Note size, shape, mobility, and tenderness (Figure 14–12).

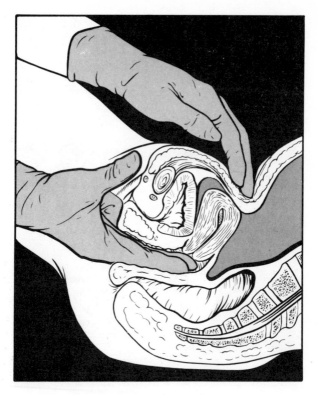

Figure 14–10. Palpation of cervix.

Rectovaginal Exam

Change gloves and lubricate index and middle finger. Insert index finger into vagina, the middle finger into rectum (Figure 14–13). Repeat maneuvers of bimanual exam with special attention to area in rectum behind cervix. Remove fingers. Use stool on glove of middle finger to perform test for occult blood (guaiac).

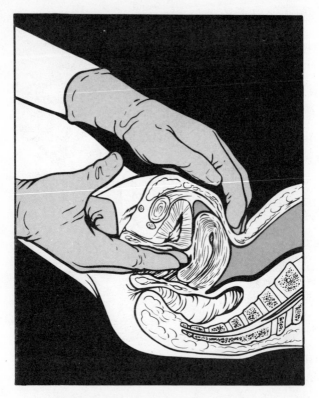

Figure 14–11. Bimanual palpation of uterus.

Recording

Normal

Normal female hair distribution. No swelling, tenderness, redness of vulva. No cysts or rectocele. Vagina pink without lesions or discharge. Cervical os closed without lesions or

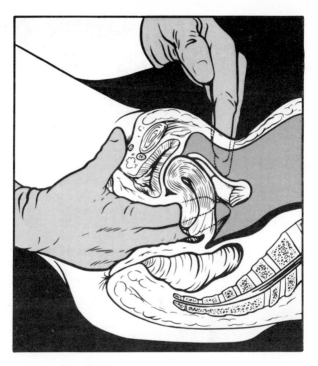

Figure 14–12. Bimanual palpation of ovaries.

erosions. Uterus small, firm, without tenderness. Ovaries palpable; no masses or tenderness. Rectal sphincter firm. Rectovaginal examination confirms findings above. Pap smears taken.

Abnormal

Normal female hair distribution. Vulva without swelling or redness. Vaginal mucosa reddened with white exudate

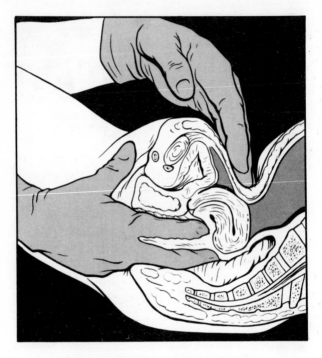

Figure 14–13. Rectovaginal examination.

present on wall. No cervical lesions or erosions. Thin, watery discharge with no odor. Uterus anterior smooth and not enlarged. Ovaries not palpated. Pap smears taken.

The patient with these abnormal findings would be at high risk for the following nursing diagnoses:

Altered skin integrity
Infection

15 | Assessment of Male Genitalia and Rectum

History Questions

Problems with urination
    Frequency, urgency, stream, nocturia, incontinence, pain
Testicular changes
    Tenderness, pain, change in size
    Self-examination practice
Evidence of hernia
    Visible bulging
Discharge from or sore on penis
Sexually transmitted diseases
    Gonorrhea, syphilis, herpes virus, scabies
    Course of illness; specific treatment, outcome
Painful sores or blisters on inner thighs, buttocks, or groin
Rectal problems
    Stool color
    Bleeding, constipation, hemorrhoids
Sexual functioning
    Activity, adjustment, changes, problems, impotence
    Number of sexual partners with high risk for HIV infection
    Frequency of testicular examination

Examination

The techniques of inspection and palpation are used to examine the male genitalia. Use of gloves by the examiner is a reasonable practice.

Patient Education
An important part of this examination is encouraging testicular self-examination. Demonstrate this technique during the examination (Figure 15–1 illustrates anatomy of the male genitalia).

Inspection and Palpation
Inspect and palpate the following structures:

Penis. Note hair distribution, size, shape, color, lesions, edema, nodules. Ask the patient to retract the prepuce and note glands for hygiene, size and placement of urethral meatus, discharge, lesions.

Scrotum. Note general size, contour, skin color (normally the left side is larger than the right). Spread walls of scrotum

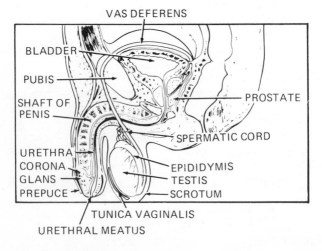

Figure 15–1. Anatomy of male genitalia.

between fingers and note lesions, nodules. Lift scrotum to inspect posterior surface. Using thumbs and forefingers compare content of each scrotal side.

Identify the testes, noting consistency, size, shape, tenderness, nodules, symmetry; identify the epididymis on the posterior surface of the testes noting symmetry, tenderness, size, shape. Grasp spermatic cord on each side at neck of scrotum, between thumb and forefinger. Palpate length of cord down to testes. Note any masses or thickening.

Transilluminate any swelling. Hold pen light behind the scrotal content. Serous fluid will transilluminate; blood and tissue will not.

Hernias

With the patient standing, inspect inguinal and femoral regions for scars, lesions, enlarged lymph nodes, hernia bulges. Ask patient to strain to accentuate bulges.

Palpate the inguinal canal by invaginating loose fold of the scrotal sac into the external inguinal ring with the fingertip. Ask the patient to strain. An indirect hernia will come down the inguinal canal and touch or tap the fingertip. A direct hernia will bulge anteriorly and push the side of the finger forward (see Figures 15–2 through 15–6 for illustrations of hernias).

Rectum

With patient standing and leaning over the examining table (for non-ambulatory patients the left lateral position with the right knee flexed is preferred), inspect the sacrococcygeal and perineal areas for inflammation, lesions, lumps. Spread the buttocks to inspect the anal area for external hemorrhoids, skin tags, rashes, scars, fissures, fistulas. Ask the patient to bear down. Note any hemorrhoids or tags. Place pad of lubricated finger over the anus and, as sphincter relaxes, insert fingertip into anal canal (see Figure 15–7).

Direct finger toward umbilicus and note sphincter tone, tenderness, irregularities. Palpate the right lateral, posterior,

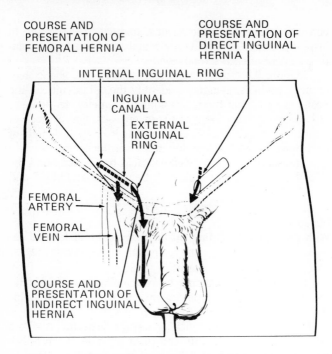

Figure 15-2. Hernias in the groin.

and left lateral surfaces, noting any irregularities. Palpate the anterior surface, identifying the lateral lobes and median sulcus of the prostate gland. Note size, shape, consistency, nodularity, tenderness. Withdraw finger from rectum and test any fecal material for occult blood (guaiac) (see Figure 15-8 for schematic view).

Recording

Normal

Normal male hair distribution. Penis circumcised; no lesions,

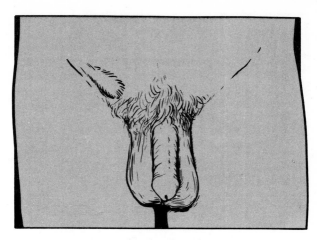

Figure 15–3. Indirect hernia (commonly seen in middle of inguinal area).

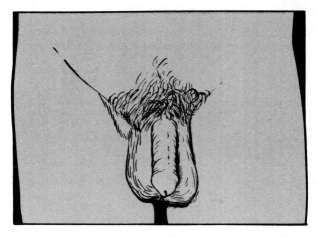

Figure 15–4. Direct hernia (commonly seen near the symphysis).

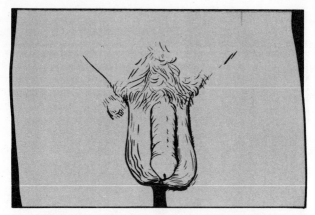

Figure 15–5. Femoral hernia (commonly seen below the inguinal ligament, near the symphysis).

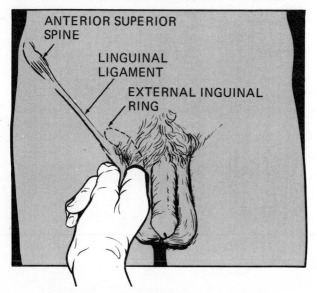

ANTERIOR SUPERIOR SPINE

LINGUINAL LIGAMENT

EXTERNAL INGUINAL RING

Figure 15–6. Palpation of the inguinal canal.

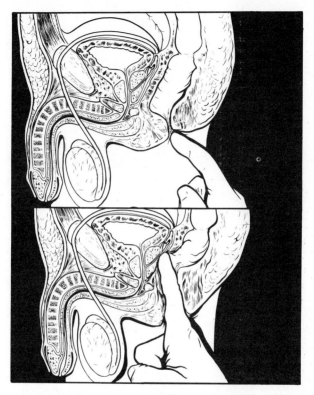

Figure 15–7. Insertion of fingertip into rectum.

inflammation, or structural alterations; urethral opening patent. Testicles descended and symmetrical without redness, masses, or tenderness. No rectal hemorrhoids, fissures, or fistulae; sphincter intact with good tone; prostate small and non-tender. Stool light brown; guaiac negative.

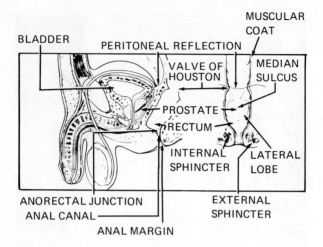

Figure 15–8. Male anus and rectum.

Abnormal

Normal pubic hair distribution. Testicles descended; no scrotal masses. Circumcised penis with two small raised vesicles on lip of circumcised fold; no penile discharge. Rectal examination elicits pain and reveals firm, enlarged, tender, boggy prostate gland. Rectal mucosa normal with no internal or external hemorrhoids. Stool brown with no visible blood; guaiac negative.

The patient with these abnormal findings would be at high risk for the following nursing diagnoses:

Altered skin integrity
Potential for altered patterns of urinary elimination

16 | Assessment of the Neurological System

History Questions*

Headaches
  Description, character, frequency, location
  Onset, duration, accompanying symptoms
  Relief, medications
  Past history, exacerbations
Vertigo, syncope
Convulsions, aura, description, frequency, triggering
  mechanism; where do they start, do they spread?
Paralysis, paresthesia, neuralgia
  Description, location, onset
Memory and orientation
  Short- and long-term
  Amnesia episodes
Visual difficulties
  Double vision, areas of blindness
  Loss of eye movement
Facial Weakness
  Drooping eyelid, cheek, mouth
Difficulty with handling saliva, drooling, problems with
  swallowing

---

*Much of the text from this portion of the physical examination is taken from E.B. Rudy, *Advanced Neurological and Neurosurgical Nursing.* C.V. Mosby Co., St. Louis, Mo., 1984.

Difficulty with head and neck movements
Problems with gait, balance
Pain in back or lower extremities
Muscle weakness or unusual muscle activity

(Figure 16–1 illustrates the main anatomical structure of the brain.)

Examination

The neurological examination is accomplished primarily through observing the patient in performing normal activities and some special maneuvers to detect deficits. The neurological examination is done near the end of the physical because many of the elements of the examination have already been performed, but an organized summary should be completed with any additional findings. The components of the neurological examination include cerebral functioning, cranial nerve

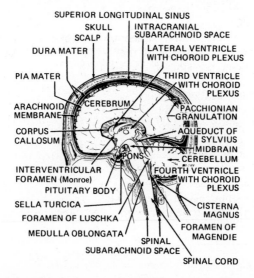

Figure 16–1. Main anatomical structure of the brain.

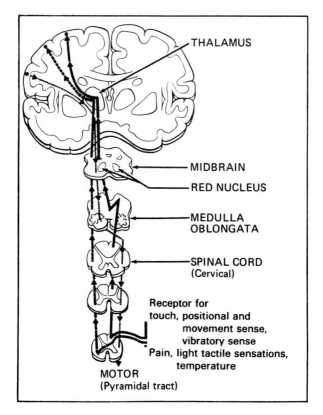

Figure 16–2. Main motor and sensory pathways.

functioning, cerebellar functioning, motor and sensory system functioning and reflexes. (Figure 16–2 shows a schematic of main motor and sensory pathways.)

Cerebral Function
Cerebral functioning can be evaluated by observing the pa-

tient's behavior throughout the interview and examination. The areas that need evaluation include:

Mental status, level of consciousness
Short-term memory; long-term memory
Emotional status, affect, and mood
Cognitive abilities, coherency, thought process, abstract reasoning
Behavior, appropriateness of responses, dress and grooming, facial expressions, speech

In most cases it is fairly easy to evaluate cerebral functioning during the history taking. Although cognitive ability is important, it is only important in terms of what is "normal" for that patient.

Patients who require a more in-depth analysis of cerebral functioning are patients with organic brain disease, or neurotic and psychotic disorders. For patients who may have these underlying problems, it is worth asking questions related to reasoning, such as explaining the proverb "Honesty is the best

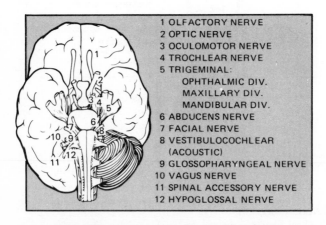

1 OLFACTORY NERVE
2 OPTIC NERVE
3 OCULOMOTOR NERVE
4 TROCHLEAR NERVE
5 TRIGEMINAL:
   OPHTHALMIC DIV.
   MAXILLARY DIV.
   MANDIBULAR DIV.
6 ABDUCENS NERVE
7 FACIAL NERVE
8 VESTIBULOCOCHLEAR (ACOUSTIC)
9 GLOSSOPHARYNGEAL NERVE
10 VAGUS NERVE
11 SPINAL ACCESSORY NERVE
12 HYPOGLOSSAL NERVE

Figure 16–3. Anatomy of origin of cranial nerves.

policy"; or asking a question that requires judgment, such as "What should you do if you are stopped by the police for going through a red light?"

Cranial Nerves

Assessment of the cranial nerves (Figure 16–3) is properly a part of the neurological examination. However, the 12 pairs of cranial nerves innervate the structures of the head and neck and are, therefore, tested in the physical examination of the head and neck. If the cranial nerve examination was not recorded after the head and neck exam, it should be completed and recorded at this time.

The cranial nerves, with the proper function and test for each nerve, are listed in Table 16–1. Each nerve is also labeled, indicating whether it has sensory or motor function or both.

Cerebellar Function

To test cerebellar function look for fine motor skills, coordination, and balance.

Coordination and Balance Tests

Finger to nose
> Ask patient to put his finger to his nose and then touch examiner's finger; repeat this maneuver rapidly several times.
> Ask patient to repeat with opposite hand.

Heel to shin
> Have patient run the heel of one foot rapidly up and down shin of opposite leg. Repeat with opposite foot.

Big toe to finger
> Have patient touch his big toe to examiner's finger, repeat rapidly several times. Repeat with opposite foot.

Rapid alternating movements
> Have patient perform rapid alternating movement with both hands. For example, touch thumb to each finger rapidly going from small finger to index finger. May

TABLE 16-1. ASSESSMENT OF CRANIAL NERVE FUNCTION

Cranial Nerve	Function	Test
I. Olfactory (S)	Smell	Identifies familiar odors such as coffee, cloves, mint, with eyes closed. Often omitted unless there is a problem
II. Optic (S)	Visual fields	Visual fields correspond to the tracts of the optic nerve and include nasal and temporal fields of both eyes. These fields of vision can be grossly evaluated by having the patient cover one eye, look straight ahead, and identify when he sees a penlight or wiggling finger. The examiner tests each visual field and then has the patient cover the other eye and repeats the test
	Visual acuity	Use Snellen eye chart or ask patient to read normal printed material. (This is only a gross evaluation.)
III. Oculomotor (M)	Pupil constriction	With penlight, check for pupil constriction in each eye and consensual constriction in opposite eye

Accommodation

Check pupil constriction as finger is moved from 3 feet away to a few inches from the eyes. Pupils dilate for distance, constrict for close vision

Movement of eye muscle (Superior Rectus, Inferior Rectus, Inferior Oblique, Medial Rectus). Up and lateral, down and lateral, up and nasally

Extraocular Eye Movements (EOM)

Three cranial nerves (III, IV, & VI) innervate the muscles of the eye and have control over coordinated eye movements. Weakness or paralysis of eye muscles is evaluated by having the patient follow the examiner's finger while holding the head still to the six cardinal directions of gaze, shown on the figure below

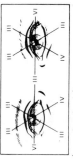

Oculomotor test by eye movements up and nasally, up and lateral, down and lateral, and nasally

Eyelid opening

Check for ptosis by evaluating position of eyelid in relation to rim of pupil

(continued)

TABLE 16-1. ASSESSMENT OF CRANIAL NERVE FUNCTION (Continued)

Cranial Nerve	Function	Test
IV. Trochlear (M)	Movement of eye muscle (Superior Oblique). Eye movement down and out, intorsion and inward rotation of eyeball	EOM (see drawing above) Tested by eye movement down and nasally
V. Trigeminal (M)	Jaw muscles and muscles of mastication	Have patient open and close jaw tightly; feel for muscle contraction
(S)	Opthalmic: Forehead, cornea Maxillary: Cheek Mandibular: Jaw, mucous membrane of mouth	Have patient identify light tactile sensation (cotton wisp) on face with eyes closed. Test corneal reflex with cotton wisp only if defect is suspected
VI. Abducens (M)	Movement of eye muscle (Lateral Rectus). Lateral movement of eyes to temporal side of head	EOM (see drawing p. 191)

VII. Facial (M)	Movement of muscles of face and scalp, eyelid closing	Have patient frown, smile, puff cheeks, close eyes tightly and resist opening
(S)	Taste anterior 2/3 tongue	Often deferred unless neurological problem. To test, have patient identify familiar taste—sugar, coffee, salt—on anterior of tongue
VIII. Acoustic (S)	Cochlear; hearing	Can be grossly evaluated by having patient repeat a whispered word or identify ticking watch. Some also use the Weber and Rinne tests to evaluate hearing (see ear exam)
	Vestibular: equilibrium	Romberg test (See description of test under cerebellar function.)
IX. Glossopharyngeal (S)	Taste: posterior half of tongue; Sensation in posterior eardrum and pharynx; Pain, touch, and temperature in pharynx and throat	Usually deferred unless neurological problem. Patient is asked to close eyes and identify familiar tastes, such as salt or sugar, on back of tongue
(M)	Muscles of pharynx	Tested with vagas (X) nerve

(continued)

TABLE 16-1. ASSESSMENT OF CRANIAL NERVE FUNCTION (Continued)

Cranial Nerve	Function	Test
X. Vagus (M) (S)	Muscles of pharynx and larynx Sensation in larynx, trachea, lungs, esophagus Slows heart, contracts bronchial muscles and produces other involuntary activity	Test these two nerves IX + X together by testing gag reflex, swallowing, and phonation. Ask patient to say "ah." Watch for symmetry of soft palate, gross deviation of uvula
XI. Spinal accessory (M)	Muscles of neck (sternocleidomastoid) and upper shoulders (trapezius)	Have patient turn head to each side against resistance of examiner's hand. Ask patient to shrug shoulders upward against resistance of examiner's hand
XII. Hypoglossal (M)	Tongue movement	Have patient protrude tongue; note tremors or deviation. Have patient push tongue against cheeks

also have patient rapidly turn hand palm up then
back of hand up and repeat several times (supination
and pronation of hand).

Romberg

Have patient stand with feet together and arms out with
eyes open. If patient loses balance, this indicates inner
ear (vestibular) problem or cerebellar ataxia. If bal-
anced with eyes open, have patient *close eyes* to test
sensory equilibrium. *Be prepared to catch patient.*

Dysfunction will be imbalance (+ Romberg).

Gait

Have patient walk in a straight line heel to toe, tandem
walking, to determine balance.

Have patient walk rapidly across floor, turn and walk
rapidly back to examining table. Observe gait characteristics.

Many conditions may produce gait disturbances that are
not related to nervous system disorders. For this
reason, terms such as *ataxic* or *spastic gate* should be
applied only at the end of the examination when the
entire picture is known. Points to observe in gait
evaluation are:

Position of the patient's head in relation to the neck and
its mobility in walking and turning.

Stance of feet, wide apart or normal distance.

Pattern of steps taken, whether the steps are short and
quick, shuffling, or wide and waddling in nature.

Presence of any swaying or staggering, and in what
direction.

Body movement during walking, whether the body
moves freely or appears "fixed."

Arm swing, whether normal or asymmetrical with one
arm moving and one arm hanging without movement.

Motor System

This portion of the neurological examination may have already
been done as part of the musculoskeletal exam. If so, do not

repeat exam; rather, refer to musculoskeletal exam.

Symmetry of muscle size (side-to-side comparison)
Look for loss of muscle mass, especially between fingers and at temporalis muscle.
Muscle tone
Look for spasticity, uncoordination, flaccidity, rigidity
Muscle strength
Test upper extremities by extensor muscles, having patient extend wrists and arms against resistance.
Test lower extremities by having patient pull heel toward buttocks while examiner provides resistance by holding onto foot. Test dorsiflexion by instructing the patient to push down and pull up with the foot against resistance from the examiner's hand.

Voluntary muscle dysfunction usually involves the pyramidal spinal tract and results in muscle weakness, whereas involuntary muscle movement usually involves the extrapyramidal spinal tracts and results in abnormal muscle movements. Table 16–2 describes some involuntary muscle movements.

Problems with muscle strength and function can be caused by:

Muscle disease
Dysfunction or problems of the neuromuscular junction
Peripheral disease (including cut motor fibers to muscles)
Spinal cord lesion or disruption
Cerebral lesion of pyramidal tract

In trying to distinguish upper motor neuron symptoms from lower motor neuron symptoms, refer to the descriptions in Table 16–3.

Sensory System Function
The sensory system is tested by having the patient identify various sensory stimuli. In a comprehensive examination all of the primary sensory functions are tested. These include tactile or light touch, superficial pain, deep pain, vibratory, position

TABLE 16-2. INVOLUNTARY MUSCLE MOVEMENTS

Type	Description
Athetosis	A slow movement of the peripheral parts of one or more limbs. These slow, rhythmic motions appear wormlike, with the wrist usually flexed and the finger hyperextended. Facial grimaces usually accompany limb movements. Voluntary movements of the affected limbs are nearly impossible. Athetosis results from damage to the area of the globus pallidus and the striate body and may be caused by birth injury or several diseases including encephalitis and tabes dorsalis (tertiary syphilis).
Ballism	Symptoms include violent, abnormal, flail-like movements of large areas of the body. For example, a leg may suddenly jerk to full flexion, or an arm may be flung upward with great force, or the body trunk may go into a sudden torsion movement. Such uncontrolled, sudden movements obviously impede walking or normal activity; however, such movements cease during sleep. Ballism or hemiballism (one sided) may result from a lesion in the subthalamic nucleus.
Chorea	Symptoms include jerky, irregular, purposeless movements of the limbs accompanied by involuntary facial twitchings. In the extreme form the patient appears engaged in a bizarre dance, thus *St. Vitus' Dance.*
Dystonia	Symptoms include distorted twisting or movement of a part or all of the body. These movements are less severe than those described as athetosis. It may be caused by toxic or infectious diseases as well as degenerative ones.

(continued)

TABLE 16-2. INVOLUNTARY MUSCLE MOVEMENTS (Continued)

Type	Description
Fascicultations	These are irregular small muscle contractions that usually are seen as a twitching or jumping muscle. While the movement causes no discomfort to the patient, it may indicate degeneration at the neuromuscular junction or anterior horn cell degeneration.
Myoclonus	This is a sudden, involuntary muscle contraction or spasm, which may involve only one muscle or a group of muscles. The muscle spasms can be severe enough to involve the entire body.
Paralysis Agitans (Parkinson's Disease)	This set of symptoms is characterized by rigidity of movement, tremors at rest, and bradykinesia (difficulty in initiating voluntary movements). Parkinson's disease results from degenerative changes in the globus pallidus and substantia nigra.
Tics	Spasmodic muscular contraction usually involving the face, head, neck, or shoulder muscles. The spasms may be tonic or clonic and may appear purposeful, such as winking the eye. Causes include degenerative changes, pressure on nerves, or may be psychogenic in nature. Tics involve the same muscle each time and can sometimes be voluntarily inhibited only to reappear later.
Tremors	A quivering, continuous, shaking movement of a part(s) of the body. Caused by alternate contractions of opposing muscles, and may be classified as involuntary, static, dynamic, kinetic, hereditary, or hysteric. The trembling motion may vary in intensity from fine to coarse, and rapid to slow; and may be present at rest or appear only upon voluntary movement.

TABLE 16-3. UPPER AND LOWER MOTOR NEURON SYMPTOMS

Upper Motor Neuron Lesion	Lower Motor Neuron Lesion
1. Spastic paralysis (knocks out inhibiting fibers to muscles)	Flaccid paralysis
2. Exaggerated deep tendon reflexes	Absence of deep tendon reflexes
3. No muscle atrophy	Atrophy of muscles
4. Positive Babinski	Normal Babinski
5. No fasciculations, cog wheel rigidity	Fasciculation due to degeneration of myoneural junction
6. Motor involvement to *opposite* side from brain lesion	Motor involvement *same* side as lesion

sense, and temperature. The examination is done with the *patient's eyes closed* and proceeds by testing corresponding body parts on each side of the body. That is, right arm to left arm, right leg to left leg. The patient is asked to compare the sensation on one side to the same sensation on the opposite side. Minimal differences are common and usually are insignificant. In general, the patient should be able to:

> interpret sensations correctly (sharp vs. dull, hot vs. cold)
> discriminate which side of the body is being stimulated
> locate on the body where the stimulus is being applied and if this is proximal or distal to the previous stimulus.

Primary Sensory Functions. (Patient's *eyes closed*.)

Tactile. Using a cotton wisp, have patient identify when (or if) sensation is felt.

Superficial Pain. Using a safety pin or paper clip, have the patient distinguish sharp from dull, increased or decreased sensations, location of sensation.

Deep Pain. Squeeze calf, biceps, or trapezius if necessary to determine the ability to identify deep pain. This is reserved for patients who lack ability to distinguish superficial pain.

Vibratory. Place tuning fork on bony prominences, beginning with distal joints first. Patient should be able to identify vibrations and locations. Test ankles, shin, knees, wrists, elbows, and shoulders. Deficits are often found in distal areas of limbs first.

Position Sense. By placing your fingers at the sides of the patient's joints, move patient's finger up and down to see if he or she can discern which way you are moving the finger. Repeat with toes.

Temperature. Occasionally you may want to know if patient can distinguish heat from cold. Use test tubes filled with water to test this function. This test is used infrequently, but may be useful since temperature sensations are carried by different sensory fibers than are vibratory sensations.

Whenever a sensory deficit is identified it should be described and, if possible, the extent of the deficit should be sketched. In this way the corresponding spinal nerve dermatome or peripheral nerve innervation can be more easily assessed.

Following the testing of primary sensory functions, testing of secondary or cortical functions is done to determine lesions in the sensory cortex or posterior columns of the spinal cord. Secondary or discriminative sensory functions combine coordination ability with the cerebral cognitive ability to interpret. Such testing is done only in patients with neurological deficits or other symptoms. Detailed testing is not necessary for routine exams.

Secondary or Cortical Sensory Functions. (Patient's *eyes closed*.)

Stereognosis. Put a familiar object such as coin or key in the patient's hand and ask him to identify it. This requires patient to "feel" the object and then figure out what it is.

Graphesthesia. Draw a number or letter of the alphabet in palm of patient's hand with a blunt pen or pencil and have patient identify it.

Point Location. Touch a point on patient's skin. Ask patient to open his eyes and point to area touched. This is useful in identifying deficits on trunk and legs.

Two-point Discrimination. Using two pins or similar objects, touch the patient's skin with both points. Find the point at which the person can no longer distinguish two points. This will be farther apart on skin areas with fewer sensory fibers and closer together in highly innervated areas. On finger pads, which are highly sensitive, the patient can normally distinguish two points as close as 2 to 3 mm apart; on the trunk or legs the points will be much farther apart.

Extinction. Stimulate a corresponding area on each side of the body. Ask the patient where he feels the sensation—normally it will be felt on both sides. An abnormal finding would be for sensation on one side to make the sensation on the opposite side extinct.

Reflexes. The reflex response is the contraction of a specific muscle when the tendon of insertion is suddenly stretched by a light tap with the finger or reflex hammer. The reflexes usually checked include the deep tendon reflexes (Table 16–4) and the superficial reflexes (Figure 16–4). The deep tendon reflexes routinely checked are the biceps, triceps, brachioradialis, patellar, and achilles.

TABLE 16-4. DEEP TENDON REFLEXES

Tendon Reflexes	Nerve Root Tested
Achilles	S_1, S_2
Patella	L_2, L_3, L_4
Biceps and Brachoradialis	C_5, C_6
Triceps	C_6, C_7, C_8

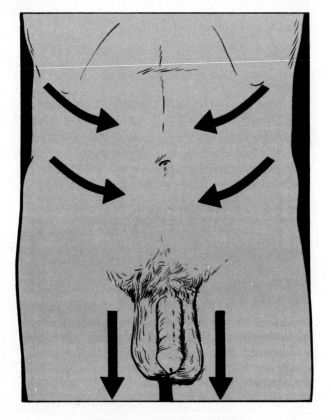

Figure 16–4. Superficial reflexes.

The grading of the muscle response is usually recorded in the following manner:

Grade 0	0	Absent
Grade 1	+	Diminished but present
Grade 2	+ +	Normal
Grade 3	+ + +	Brisker than normal
Grade 4	+ + + +	Hyperactive (clonus)

Recording

Normal
Alert and oriented, appropriate behavior and responses, memory intact.

Cranial nerves:

I	Identifies peppermint (often deferred)
II	Able to read newsprint at 12 inches, 20/20 both eyes by Snellen chart, fields of vision normal by gross confrontation (see eye exam)
III, IV, VI	Extraocular movements (EOM) intact, no ptosis, pupils equal, round, react to light and accommodate (PERRLA)
V	Facial sensation intact, clenches jaw without weakness
VII	Moves facial muscles without weakness, face symmetrical (taste deferred)
VIII	Hearing intact (see ear)
IX, X	Phonation, swallowing, gag reflex intact (taste deferred)
XI	Moves head and shrugs shoulders without weakness or difficulty
XII	Tongue movement normal

(*Note:* In many cases it is acceptable to record CN II through XII as grossly intact.)

Able to perform alternating movements without difficulty; gait, balance and coordination normal. Romberg negative. Muscles symmetrical, no weakness or atrophy noted. Sensory system intact for light touch, superficial pain and vibrations (Table 16–5).

Reflexes:

Abnormal

Alert and oriented, appropriate behavior and responses, memory intact. Cranial nerves II through XII grossly intact. Unable to perform rapid alternating movement; resting tremors present in both hands. Gait is wide-based with short shuffling steps; arms are riding at side with walking. No muscle atrophy noted, sensory system intact for light touch, superficial pain and vibrations.

Reflexes:

The patient with these abnormal findings would be at high risk for the following nursing diagnosis:

Impaired physical mobility

TABLE 16-5. SUPERFICIAL REFLEXES

Tendon Reflexes	Nerve Root Tested
Upper Abdominal reflex (stroke ↑ upper abdomen, umbilicus pulls to stimulated side.)	T_7, T_8, T_9
Lower Abdominal Reflex (stroke ↓ lower abdomen, umbilicus pulls to stimulated side.)	T_{10}, T_{11}
Cremasteric reflex (stroke inner thigh, scrotum goes ↑)	T_{12}, L_1, L_2
Plantar (Babinski) (with sharp object stroke lateral sole of foot from heel to ball of foot and across ball of foot.)	S_1, S_2 ↑ A positive response is dorsiflexion of the big toe with fanning of the other toes and shows pyramidal tract disease.

17 | Assessment of the Pediatric Patient

HEALTH HISTORY

The pediatric health history is very important as it provides opportunity to interview both the child and the parent(s) in order to gather pertinent information about the health status of the child, including pattern of growth and development, relationships with others, and specific child care. While the pediatric history is an adaptation of the adult health history, it incorporates areas specific to the child. It is for this reason that the following complete pediatric health history is outlined:

IDENTIFYING DATA

Name
Sex
Address (child and parents or guardian)
Telephone numbers
Race
Country of origin if recent immigrant
Primary language
Significant characteristics—skin color and the geographic origin of child's ancestors
Adolescent—religion, marital status, number of children, presence of chronic disease

CHIEF COMPLAINT

This will often only be noted as Well Child Care or Health Maintenance for management of routine preventive care.

Common complaints include "checkup," "baby shots," "earache," "flus," "school problems," "vomiting." Duration of the symptoms that are the cause of the complaint should be noted.

PAST HEALTH

Birth history (including prenatal history)
Condition at birth
Neonatal period
Early infancy
Childhood—adolescent health
    Common childhood diseases
    Serious illnesses
    Surgical procedures
    Accidents and injuries
    Allergies
    Immunizations

PATIENT PROFILE

Current life situation
Household members with relationship to child
Physical characteristics of home
    Location
    Neighborhood
    Water supply
    Sewage system

Primary care-givers
School attending
  All educational settings
  Address
  Grade
  Teacher's name
Economic situation
Agencies involved with child and family

DEVELOPMENTAL HISTORY

Have parents answer following questions:

How would you describe your child to a person who does not know him?
Do you know of specific weaknesses or problems your child has?
What do you consider the most enjoyable things about your child?
What do you consider the most difficult things about your child?
How does this child compare with his or her siblings?
Describe quality of child's relationship with the parents, siblings, and others in the household.
How is child disciplined?

HABITS

Feedings
  Difficulties
  Patterns
Sleeping arrangements

Naps
Number of hours
Toileting
Age of toilet training
Frequency
Enuresis
Day-time wetting

CHILDHOOD RELATIONSHIPS

Adjustments to school setting
Relationship with parents and siblings
Relationships with peers and teachers
Separation anxiety
Attention span
Content and quality of play

LANGUAGE AND COMMUNICATION

Infant and Toddler

Single and combined vowel sounds
Simple consonants
Jargon
Specific words and phrases
Name body parts
Follow simple directions
Describe pictures in book

Older Child

Quality of enunciation
Some grammatically correct sentences
Presence of stuttering

Beginning ability to read and write depending upon age in
   school

Adolescent

Ease in speaking with peers and parents
Ability to share concerns and interests
Ability to respond to questions relating directly to habits,
   responsibilities, and discipline
Speaking and writing skills

MOTOR SKILLS

Fine Motor

Thumb-finger prehension (use of hand muscles for ma-
   nipulating small objects)
Hand-age coordination
   grasp, hold, release objects
Aptitude for completing tasks (buttoning)

Gross Motor

Large muscle use of limbs and trunk
Age-appropriate skills (running, jumping)

ADAPTIVE ABILITY

Evaluate performance of structural tasks (copy geometric
   figures)
Knowledge of colors
Ability to complete age-appropriate puzzles

FAMILY MEDICAL HISTORY

Diseases with strong genetic component
Diseases that are highly infectious
Pedigree of three generations

REVIEW OF SYSTEMS

General state of health and growth—ask parent to describe child's health status. Child over the age of 10 can answer this question.

Diet
Record if child is receiving adequate nutrition: describe any specific diet.

Skin
Dry or oily, temperature, color, and texture; rashes, acne (especially in adolescents).

Hair
Excessive growth of fine hair, texture, hirsutism.

Nails
Evidence of biting; abnormalities.

Head and Neck
Headache, pain, injuries, facial symmetry, neck stiffness, pain, masses.

Ears
Infections, pain, discharge, hearing, tinnitus.

Eyes
Vision problems, strabismus, infections, pain, injury. Date of last vision test, results. If child wears glasses determine reason, when prescribed, and if vision improved.

Nose
Breathing problems, septum, drainage, sinus pain, nose-bleeds.

Mouth and Throat
Sore throat, sores in mouth, cracked lips, chewing or swallowing problems, hoarseness, dental care, pacifier, thumb or finger sucking.

Breasts
Changes, pain, discharge, infections, masses, nipple abnormality. In prepubescent girl: soreness, beginning development, asymmetry in size and shape during pubertal growth. In the adolescent boy: gynecomastia.

Respiratory Tract
Breathing problems, cough, sputum consistency, amount, color, hemoptysis, wheezing, asthma, chest pain, any infections including pneumonia.

Cardiovascular System
History of murmurs, shortness of breath, cyanosis with exertion, feeding problems, excessive crying, irritability, vomiting, squatting behavior; chest pain with exertion.

Gastrointestinal Tract
Vomiting (frequency; projectile) frequency of stool describing color, form, consistency, odor, mucous, any blood or parasites; abdominal pain, food intolerance, unusual flatus, pica.

Urinary Tract
Habits, urine color, quality of stream, quantity, urgency; dysuria, polyuria, enuresis; edema of forehead and hands.

Genital Tract
Male—Penile pain or discharge; testicular pain, swelling, or masses, other scrotal masses, rashes, or hernias, changes in genital size and appearance of pubic hair in the adolescent. If

adolescent is sexually active, history of sexually transmitted disease and use of contraceptives.

Female—Prepuberty: Vaginal discharge or itching; knowledge of pubertal changes and menstruation. Pubertal: Menarche date and age, frequency cycle, regularity, quality of flow, dysmenorrhea, date of last period, vaginal discharge, determine attitude toward menstrual cycle.

Musculoskeletal System
Muscle, bone, joint pain; swelling, redness, tenderness, range of motion, stiffness deformity.

Nervous System
Weakness, headache, convulsions, ataxia, paresthesia, fainting, speech problems, dizziness.

Hematopoietic System
Pallor, unusual bleeding, nosebleeds, blood in stools, bruising, enlarged lymph nodes, transfusions.

Travel
Into any areas where infectious diseases are known to be endemic.

Pets
Significant for infectious disease and allergic disorders.

Psychological Disorders
Mood or affect changes; depressions; difficult relationships with parents, peers, authority figures; nervousness; change in eating behavior; phobias; sudden change in school performance.

PHYSICAL EXAMINATION

The physical examination of children who are at various stages of growth and development necessitates that the examiner develop skill in approaching and communicating with each child. The procedure may be more easily accomplished for the child receiving well child care than for the child who is ill. To negate normal fear, the examination may be done while the child sits on the mother's lap. If, however, the child needs to be placed on the examining table, the examiner should be at eye level in order to establish mutual trust.

In many areas, the physical examination of the child is similar to, if not the same as, that of the adult. Only those areas where the child's examination differs from the adult are included in the following section.

SKIN AND INTEGUMENT

Infancy and Childhood

Assessment of the child's integument requires answers to questions regarding nutrition, family allergies, presence of pets, health of family, playmates, and family hygiene and habits. The child's skin is inspected for color, texture, turgor, and lesions. The skin of infants and children differs from that of adults. The infant's skin appears soft, smooth, and almost transparent. The epidermis is thin, poorly developed, and susceptible to irritation and infection. Sweating is scanty or even absent. In black infants, deeper pigmentation is seen in the nailbeds and the scrotum.

Nevus flammeus, in the form of small, red papular patches, may be visible over the infant's occiput, forehead, and upper eyelids. This is of no clinical significance and usually disappears before one year of age. *Café-au-lait spots,* in the form of small, macular, bright brown stains, may also be visible in one or two patches. Numerous patches, however, are suggestive of *fibromas* or *neurofibromatoses* and require further attention. *Dehydrated* infants have loose, extra skin at the calf. It is for this reason that skin turgor is best evaluated by palpating this area. There are numerous disorders of the child's skin. Some of these are included in Table 17–1. Commonly occurring child-hood infectious diseases that produce rashes are included in Table 17–2.

Awareness of the significance of bruises is of paramount importance in examining the child's skin. In the normal, active child, *ecchymoses* and *hematomas*, especially on the extremities, are common. If, however, parents report weakness and fatigue, and the appearance of spontaneous bruising, blood dyscrasias such as *leukemia* and *hemophilia* are suspected. Battered children will also present with bruises and hematomas, but the history will describe unusual events and circumstances that need further explanation and investigation.

The nails of the child are inspected for color, trauma, nail biting, lesions, infections of the cuticle, and clubbing. The head and hair are inspected for signs of lice, mites, or ticks. Normally, from birth to puberty, heavy amounts of hair are found on the scalp, eyebrows, and lashes. Deviation in this hair growth pattern needs investigation.

Adolescence

After the first year of life, there is little change in the normal child's skin until the onset of puberty. At this time, there is development of the sweat and sebaceous glands and the production of hormones that affect skin and hair. Pubic and axillary hair begins to grow. Androgen levels increase, stimulating sebaceous glands to secrete large amounts of sebum that clog hair follicle openings. Common skin problems of the adolescent are acne, warts, atopic dermatitis, scabies, and pityriasis rosea. Contact dermatitis from cosmetics and jewelry, and fungal infections, especially from tinea pedia, are also common occurrences. The seriousness of acne vulgaris in the adolescent cannot be overestimated. Even mild acne affects self-concept and self-confidence essential for the establishment of new, mutual relationships and friendships. The first stage of acne consists of blackheads that develop into superficial and deep papules found on the forehead, chin, and cheeks and extending on the back, shoulders, and chest. When pustules

TABLE 17-1. SKIN DISORDERS THAT OCCUR DURING CHILDHOOD

Disorder	Age	Manifestations and Considerations
Diaper rash	Infant	*Mild:* Simple chafing to mild-erythematous macular areas *Severe:* Bright red papules with open ulcers Infections with staphylococci, *Candida albicans*, or streptococci organisms may result
Eczema	Infant	Scaliness on cheeks, behind ears, knees, and elbows, often associated with allergic reaction to cow's milk
Seborrhea, dermatitis, or cradle cap	Infant	Flakiness on the scalp over the fontanelles
Milia Rubra (Transient heat rash)	Infant	Macular rash on the face, neck, trunk, and diaper area
Intertrigo	Infant	Raw, denuded areas from rubbing of skin surfaces in moist body areas
Impetigo	All ages	Pustules filled with yellowish exudate, often crusted over, around the mouth and on the hands
Ringworm	All ages	Rash in circular pattern with scaliness
Erythema nodosum	Preschool and school	Painful, tender, reddened nodules 2–4 cm in diameter along the leg or ulnar surface of the arms, seen in children with rheumatoid arthritis
Erythema marginatum	Preschool and school	Circular reddened areas, 1 or 2 cm, with concrete borders, seen in children with rheumatic fever

TABLE 17-2. INFECTIOUS DISEASES WITH RASHES THAT OCCUR DURING EARLY CHILDHOOD

Disease	Transmission	Incubation Period	Clinical Manifestations	Rash
Chicken pox (Varicella)	Direct contact; droplet, contaminated objects	2–3 weeks	Slight fever, malaise, anorexia for first 24 hours, lymphadenopathy, temperature irritability from pruritus	Highly pruritic; first macule, then papules and vesicles. Lesions break and form crusts. Centripetal, spreading to face and proximal extremities but sparse on distal limbs
Erythema Infectiosum (Fifth disease probably virus)	Infection persons- direct contact or droplet	6–14 days	None—No lymphadenopathy	"Slapped face" appearance from rash on cheeks which disappears in 1–4 days followed by maculopapular red spots on upper and lower extremities that may last for a week

				or more; rash subsides but may reappear with irritation from the sun or friction
Roseola (Exanthem)	Unknown Limited to children 6 months to 2 years of age.	Unknown	Persistent high fever for 3–4 days in child who appears well. Precipitous drop in fever to normal with appearance of rash	Discrete rose-pink macules or maculopapules appearing on trunk, then spreading to neck, face and extremities; nonpruritic; fades on pressure; lasts for 1–2 days
Rubeola (Measles)	Direct contact with droplets of infected person	10–20 days	Prodromal fever, malaise, cough, conjunctivitis, Koplik spots (small irregular red spots with a bluish white center) on the buccal mucosa opposite the	3–4 days after prodromal stage, erythematous maculopapular eruption on face appears and spreads downward; after 3–4 days rash becomes brown

(continued)

TABLE 17-2. INFECTIOUS DISEASES WITH RASHES THAT OCCUR DURING EARLY CHILDHOOD (Continued)

Disease	Transmission	Incubation Period	Clinical Manifestations	Rash
			molars, anorexia, generalized lymphadenopathy	with fine desquamation
Rubella (German Measles)	Direct contact with infected persons; indirect by articles freshly contaminated with nasopharyngeal secretions, feces or urine	14–21 days	Prodromal stage absent in children, present in adolescents and adults. Low-grade fever, headache, malaise, anorexia, sore throat, cough, lymphadenopathy, which subsides one day after rash appears	Appears first on face and spreads rapidly to neck, arms, trunk, and legs. Body is covered in one day with pinkish red maculopapular rash. Disappears way it came in 3 days

and cysts form, scarring results. Adolescents with severe acne are always referred to a dermatologist.

The skin is also inspected for scars, needle tracks, and bruises. If these are found, additional history data are required for evaluation, treatment, and follow-up.

Pallor in the adolescent female is quite common and may indicate a low hemoglobin resulting from poor diet habits. Any suspicion of true anemia, however, is confirmed through laboratory data. Because infectious mononucleosis and hepatitis are also common in this age group, suspicion of jaundice or generalized adenopathy is investigated thoroughly.

HEAD AND NECK

Infancy and Childhood

The greatest circumference of the infant's head is measured and recorded regularly during the first year of life (Figure 17–1 lists normal measurements.) The head is observed for control, movements, and position. After the age of 3 months there should be no head lag and infant can sit propped. Auscultation for bruits is not performed until after the age of 6, as normal bruits are present over the temporal area until that age. The thyroid, trachea, and lymph nodes of the neck are palpated following the procedures used in examining the adult. Lymph node enlargement occurs readily in children with infections. Discrete, shotty, nontender, cool nodes are normal findings and usually indicate previous infections. Large, warm, tender, or isolated nodes, as well as lymphadenopathy, require referral to a physician.

Face

The face is inspected for symmetry, distribution of hair, size of mandible, and paralysis. Facial paralysis is best discerned when the child cries or smiles, which increases the asymmetry. Abnormal or unusual facies may suggest a chromosomal abnormality, as seen in the child with Down syndrome.

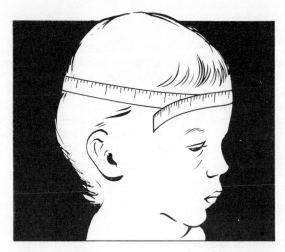

Birth	~35 cm	12 mo	~46 cm
6 mo	~43 cm	2 yr	~48 cm
9 mo	~45 cm	3 yr	~50 cm

Figure 17–1. Measurement of the infant's head at its greatest circumference.

Mouth

The lips are inspected for color, evidence of lip biting or chewing. Breath odor is noted along with the number, color, and condition of teeth. Eruption of primary teeth occurs earlier in boys than girls, whereas permanent eruption occurs earlier in girls. The sequence of tooth eruption is important and should be evaluated carefully (Figure 17–2). Excessive bottle feeding and a high carbohydrate diet increase dental caries in children. Tooth brushing should start at the time of the first dental visit at the age of 2½ to 3 years. The gums and buccal

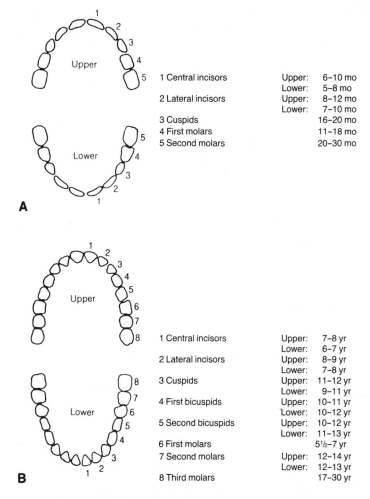

Figure 17–2. A. Timetable for eruption of deciduous teeth. **B.** Timetable for eruption of permanent teeth. *(Data from Merenstein G. B., Kaplan D. W., Rosenberg A. A. Handbook of Pediatrics, 16th ed. Appleton & Lange, Norwalk CT, 1990.)*

mucosa are inspected. A dark line at the gum margin is normally present in black children. The condition of the tongue may indicate infection or allergy and the tongue is inspected for size, color, condition, and movement.

Throat

The throat is inspected for color and condition of tonsils, presence and movement of the uvula, and color of the pharyngeal mucosa. The nature of the cry indicates laryngeal status and may herald central nervous system problems as well. Examination of the throat is unpleasant for the child, and skill by the examiner is needed to accomplish pharyngeal observation in one quick glance.

The cooperative older child will not require the use of a tongue depressor and will allow more time for throat assessment.

Nose

The external nose is inspected for shape, symmetry, nasal flaring, discharge, skin lesions, insertion of foreign body, or the allergic crease. The internal assessment includes condition of the septum and turbinates, color of mucosa, evidence of trauma, foreign bodies, and hemorrhage. The frontal and maxillary sinuses are palpated and percussed in children over the age of 6 for edema and tenderness. The maxillary sinuses are percussed directly for evidence of air-filled cavities (Figure 17–3).

Adolescence

Physical examination of the adolescent's head, neck, and face is similar to that of the adult with few exceptions. Careful palpation for evidence of bleeding is performed if there is history of acute head injury. Adolescent athletes may have limitations in neck mobility following injury, necessitating careful follow-up. Should fever and malaise accompany the lack of mobility, meningitis should be suspected and the patient referred to a physician.

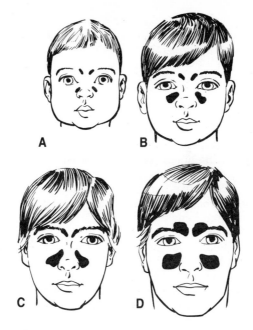

Figure 17–3. Development of the frontal and maxillary sinuses. **A.** Early infancy. **B.** Early childhood. **C.** Adolescence. **D.** Adulthood.

Mouth

Dental caries are a major problem in adolescence. Frequent dental examinations are encouraged, along with reminders that oral hygiene is very important. When braces are worn, dental examinations are essential to negate the formation of plaque and decay underneath them.

Nose

The prominent or distorted nose poses a major problem for the teenager. When the problem exists, referral to a specialist should be made. Rhinoplasty procedures are common among adolescents and positive personality changes have been reported following repair of the nose.

EYE

Infancy and Childhood

Vision in the infant can be determined grossly when the tracking of a bright light or toy is achieved at about the age of 6 weeks. Direct and consensual pupillary reaction to light is further evidence that the infant can see. Inspection of ocular movement at this age often reveals intermittent and alternating convergent strabismus and this is quite common. If, however, divergent, persistent, or unilateral strabismus is present, referral to an ophthalmologist is necessary to prevent chronic, untreated strabismus, which can lead to blindness.

Inspection of the eyes is best accomplished by holding the infant upright, with the head in mid-line, and slowly rotating the infant's body in one direction. The infant's eyes will follow the direction of rotation. When rotation ceases the infant's eyes look in the opposite direction, which is normal. The ophthalmoscope light will elicit a red reflex when it is 8–12 inches from the eye. In the Caucasion infant, the reflex is red whereas in the black infant it is orange.

The infant by 1 month can see small objects and by 2 months rough outlines and follow moving fingers. By 6 months, the infant can focus for short periods but is far-sighted.

Funduscopic examination should be performed on all infants after the age of 2 months if possible. It is helpful if the baby is held by a parent in either the lap or shoulder position. While the method of funduscopic examination is similar to that of the adult, lid retraction may be necessary. Findings are also similar to the adult except that the optic disc is paler, the peripheral vessels are not well developed, and the foveal light reflection is absent.

Visual screening for the child over 2 years of age is of paramount importance to detect amblyopia ex anopsia, reduced vision in a normal eye produced by disuse. There is disconjugate fixation, and the optic cortex suppresses one of the two images it receives in order to avoid diplopia. Therefore, one eye becomes "lazy," stops functioning to its maximum capacity and that eye's visual acuity is reduced markedly due to suppression of foveal vision. Improvement in this condition is unlikely if treatment is not started before the child is 6 years old.

The two most common causes of amblyopia ex anopsia are strabismus, a misalignment of each eye's optic axis, and anisometropia, where one eye has a refractive error 1.5 diopters or more greater than the other. Two accurate tests that screen for eye muscle weakness and visual acuity caused by these conditions are the Hirschberg test and the Cover-Uncover test.

Specifically, the *Hirschberg test* and the *Cover–Uncover test* may be used to detect muscle weakness causing one eye to deviate inwardly (esotropia) or outwardly (exotropia). To perform the Hirschberg test, the examiner looks for the corneal light reflex with the patient's eyes fixed first in the mid-line position and then to the left and right position. If the light reflex is visualized at the same corneal location bilaterally, no muscle weakness exists. If, however, deviation in corneal light reflection is present, strabismus is suspected.

The *Cover–Uncover test* (Figure 17–4) is more sophisticated than the Hirschberg test. This simple test consists of the following steps:

1. Have child fixate on an attractive object.
2. Cover left eye with an occluder (such as a paper cup or paper disc) and observe the right eye. (It should *not* move or change position to view the object.)
3. Remove the occluder from the left eye and again observe the right eye. (It should not jerk back into position. If no movements are seen, the eye is straight.)

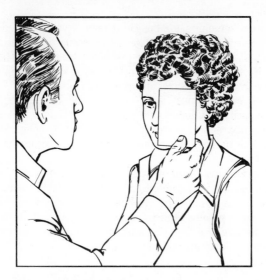

Figure 17–4. The cover–uncover test.

The test is repeated on the right eye. To detect more subtle changes, the test can be repeated in both eyes in all fields of gaze.

Normal visual acuity for the child over 3 years of age is tested using the Snellen chart (illiterate E). The child uses his or her hands and fingers to indicate in which position the "legs" of the E are pointed. Normal visual acuity for children ages 2 to 3 ranges from 12/30 to 15/30; ages 3 to 4 from 15/30 to 20/30.

Visual field testing is best accomplished by having the child sit on the parent's lap with the parent gently holding the child's head in a straightforward position. Small objects or toys are moved into the child's visual field by the examiner, following the same procedure as that of the adult.

Color blindness is more common in boys than in girls. After the age of 4, simple color screening tests can be performed such as asking the child to distinguish various colored objects or finger-tracing numbers on color vision graphs.

Children who complain of eye strain require a complete ophthalmoscopic examination, which includes pupillary dilation with mydriatic drops. If eye glasses are prescribed, the child will need assistance in adjusting to the corrective lenses.

Adolescence

The procedure for examining the eyes of the adolescent is the same as for the adult. Frequent eye examinations are necessary for this age group as myopia is a common occurrence. When myopia is present, increased demands for reading and studying produce eye strain, which necessitates corrective prescription lenses. Today, many teenagers wear contact lenses without problems, but there is continued need for encouraging proper lens hygiene, proper time use, and prevention of corneal abrasion.

EAR

Infancy and Childhood

Examination of the ears is more important for the child than for the adult because the immature structure of the child's ear makes it more prone to infection. The external ear and mastoid areas are inspected for deformity, clefts, cysts, and the position of the ears. The top of the ear should be on a horizontal line with the inner and outer canthus of the eye. During otoscopic examination the child should be held by the parent or placed in a prone position on the examining table with the external ear canal directed downward. The largest speculum is gradually inserted with caution to avoid discomfort. Because the child's ear canal is normally directed upward, the ear is pulled down and backward to permit inspection of the tympanic membrane. One finger rests against the head so that sudden movements will not cause injury. The canal is inspected for patency, color, and cerumen accumulation. The light reflex is diffused in infants. Dilation of the blood vessels in the middle ear of the crying child should not be mistaken for inflammation.

Pneumatic otoscopy is used to examine the ears of the infants and children who have symptoms of earache and/or ear infection. For this procedure, the examiner observes the tympanic membrane as pressure is increased or decreased in the external auditory canal. This is accomplished by introducing and removing air from the canal by applying positive and negative pressures with a bulb or by blowing and sucking on a rubber tube attached to the otoscope (Figures 17–5 and 17–6).

Hearing in infants is assessed by observing a blinking of the eyes in response to a sudden sharp noise. For older children, the whisper of simple commands at a distance of 8 feet is used. A complete screening test with an audiometer should be done on all children with any question of hearing difficulty before they begin school. Evaluation of hearing on a regular basis is essential.

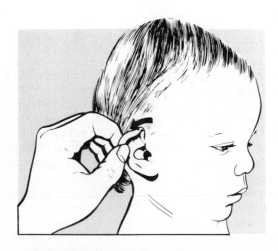

Figure 17–5. Ear position for otoscopy of infant.

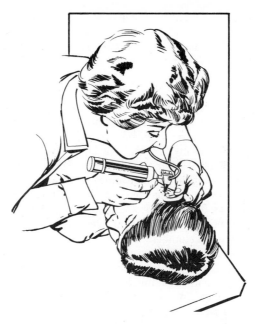

Figure 17–6. Pneumatic otoscopy in young children.

Adolescent

The adolescent's ears are examined in the same manner as the adult's.

BREASTS

Infancy and Childhood

The breasts of infants and children, male and female, before the age of puberty, consist only of branching ducts in fibrous tissue. Because there is no tissue growth until the teen years, the breast examination at this age is of no clinical significance. It is not uncommon for newborns to have engorged breasts due to transfer of maternal hormones. This will disappear in 1 to 2 months and is of no consequence.

Adolescence

It is during early adolescence that breast tissue begins to develop and mature. The young girl may complain of soreness and tingling in one or both breasts and asymmetry of the breasts is not uncommon. It is at this time of beginning breast development that the importance of the self-breast examination should be explained and encouraged. Young girls may be very self-conscious during the discussion of breast examination as well as the actual examination itself. The examiner should be especially sensitive to the needs of the young patient at this stage in development. For older adolescents the breast examination is the same as in the adult.

The male adolescent's breasts should be examined in the same manner as in the adult male. Some increase in breast tissue may appear in early adolescence in males, but overt gynecomastia requires referral for evaluation.

THORAX AND LUNGS

Infancy and Childhood

The chest is inspected for shape, symmetry, retraction, and circumference. The infant's chest is almost round, with the antero-posterior diameter as great as the transverse diameter. The chest circumference is the same or slightly less than the head circumference until 2 years of age. Respiratory activity is diaphragmatic with a simultaneous drawing in of the lower thorax and protrusion of the abdomen on inspiration and the reverse on expiration. This is referred to as paradoxical breathing. Palpation and tactile fremitus may be performed while the child is crying. Percussion of the chest may be done using the direct or indirect method and the percussion note will be hyperresonant throughout. The bell or small diaphragm is used for auscultating the child's chest. In the infant, breath sounds are much louder and harsher than the adult because of the thinness of the chest wall. In early and late childhood they remain the same except the respiratory patterns are more regular and the child can cooperate in the examination. Breath sounds are rarely absent in the infant or child because of the small size of the thorax, resulting in easy transmission of sounds.

Adolescence

The thorax and lungs are examined as in the adult. Respiratory infections and asthma are common occurrences in this age group.

CARDIOVASCULAR

Infancy and Childhood

Before beginning the examination of the young child's heart, look for other physical symptoms that may herald heart disease, then identify major peripheral pulses, the apical pulse, and finally auscultate for heart sounds and murmurs.

Presenting physical findings that could indicate heart problems include poor weight gain, poor feeding pattern, delayed development, clubbing of the fingers or toes (usually not present before 3 months of age), labored or rapid respirations, cyanosis, tachycardia, venous enlargement, and hepatic engorgement (more than 2 cm below the costal margin). These findings may also be present in the infant with "respiratory distress," infections, and central nervous system injuries, making diagnosis difficult; prompt referral for proper diagnosis and medical treatment is of prime importance.

Major peripheral pulses should be palpated with particular attention given to the femoral pulse in this age group as absent or severely diminished pulses may indicate coarctation of the aorta.

The apical impulse is often visible at the level of the 4th interspace until the age of 7 years, when with growth it is found best at the 5th interspace. The apical pulse is located to the left of the MCL before age 4; at the MCL between the ages 4 to 6; and to the right of the MCL after age 7. In palpating the apical pulse, a heaving or thrusting precordium should be taken as a possible sign of a cardiac problem.

If possible, the child's heart should be auscultated in the sitting, lying, and left lateral decubitus positions. Owing to the thinness of the chest wall, the heart sounds are louder, higher pitched, and have a shorter duration. S_1 is louder than S_2 at the apex and S_2 is louder than S_1 in the pulmonic area. Physiological splitting of the S_2 at the pulmonic area is present in most children. An S_3, or extra heart sound, is present in one-fourth to one-third of all children. As noted in the exam of the adult heart, an S_3 is not considered pathological until after the age of 40. Also, sinus arrhythmia is a common finding in children.

Because so many children develop murmurs, the differentiation between pathological and non-pathological murmurs is extremely important. Congenital cardiac abnormalities may be identifed at birth because of characteristic heart murmurs often accompanied by severe cyanosis and rapid respirations. However, some forms of congenital heart lesions do not cause impressive murmurs in the newborn period, so that severe heart problems may not be identified until later examinations. Although the description of heart murmurs receives a great deal of attention in diagnosing congenital heart disease in children, it is often difficult to distinguish a pathological murmur from an innocent murmur in a child. Innocent murmurs are characterized as systolic, of short duration, poorly transmitted, heard best lying down, and of grade 1 or 2 (out of 6) intensity. Innocent murmurs are present in a large percentage of children who are otherwise healthy. However, any murmur should make the examiner look more carefully for other signs of cardiac problems. If any additional symptoms are present or any question remains, a referral is indicated.

Some of the more common congenital cardiac abnormalities are presented on the following pages. (See also Tables

17–3 and 17–4 for heart and respiratory rates for the pediatric patient.)

CONGENITAL HEART ABNORMALITIES*

General signs and symptoms suggesting cardiac problems:

Infants	**Children**
1. Dyspnea	1. Dyspnea
2. Difficulty with feeding	2. Poor physical development
3. Stridor or choking spells	3. Decreased exercise tolerance
4. Pulse rate over 200	4. Recurrent respiratory infections
5. Recurrent respiratory infections	5. Heart murmur and thrill
6. Failure to gain weight	6. Cyanosis
7. Heart murmurs	7. Squatting
8. Cyanosis	8. Clubbing of fingers and toes
9. Cerebral-vascular accidents	9. Elevated blood pressure
10. Anoxic attacks	

Figures 17–7A through J illustrate various heart defects.

Adolescence

The cardiac examination of the adolescent parallels that of the adult. Evaluation of peripheral pulses and blood pressure should be included in the cardiac exam. The apical pulse is usually at the 5th ICS of the MCL, as in the adult. Physiological splitting of S_2 and an extra sound, S_3, are normal findings in

---

Source: General signs and symptoms of congenital heart abnormalities. Ross Laboratories, Columbus, Ohio, Division of Abbott Laboratories.

TABLE 17-3. HEART RATE VARIATIONS FOR THE PEDIATRIC CLIENT

Age	Average Range	Average Rate
Birth	90–190	140
First 6 months	80–180	130
6–12 months	75–155	115
1–2 years	70–150	110
2–6 years	68–138	103
6–10 years	65–125	95
10–14 years	55–115	85

(From Bates B. *A Guide to Physical Examination and History Taking.* Philadelphia, J.B. Lippincott, 1987)

this age group. Innocent murmurs can occasionally be identified in the teenager, but for the most part, murmurs should not be present. Generally, any murmur of this age is worth referral for further workup.

ABDOMEN

Infancy and Childhood
In infants the abdomen is protuberant, due to their poorly developed musculature. Infants are prone to umbilical hernias,

TABLE 17-4. RESPIRATORY RATES FOR CHILDREN

Age	Respiratory Rate
Newborn	30–50
6 mo	20–30
2 yr	20–30
Adolescent	12–20

(From Alexander M.M. and Brown M.S. *Pediatric Physical Diagnosis for Nurses.* New York, McGraw-Hill, 1974 p. 121)

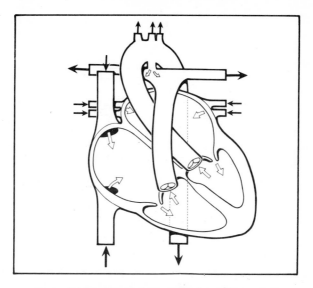

Figure 17–7A. Patent ductus arteriosus. The patent ductus artiosus is a vascular connection that, during fetal life, shortcircuits the pulmonary vascular bed and directs blood from the pulmonary artery to the aorta. Functional closure of the ductus normally occurs soon after birth. If the ductus remains patent after birth, the direction of blood flow in the ductus is reversed by the higher pressure in the aorta.

ventral hernias, and diastasis recti, all of which can be detected when the infant cries. These usually disappear the first year of life. Auscultation of the infant's abdomen should reveal metallic tinkling sounds every 20 to 30 seconds. Palpation is performed by holding the infant's legs flexed at the knees and hips with one hand, and palpating with the other. The liver edge, spleen tip, bladder, and descending colon along with inguinal lymph nodes are often palpable.

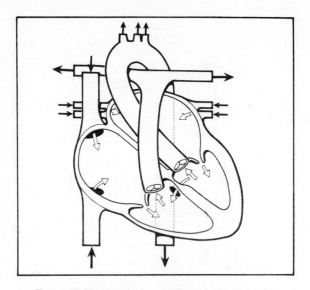

Figure 17–7B. Ventricular septal defects. A ventricular septal defect is an abnormal opening between the right and left ventricles. Ventricular septal defects vary in size and may occur in either the membranous or muscular portion of the ventricular septum. Because of higher pressure in the left ventricle, a shunting of blood from the left to right ventricle occurs during systole. If pulmonary vascular resistance produces pulmonary hypertension, the shunt of blood is then reversed from the right to the left ventricle, with cyanosis resulting.

Protuberance of the abdomen may persist throughout childhood when the child is standing on his or her feet (see Figure 17–8). It should, however, disappear when the child lies down. Light superficial palpation of the abdomen in all quadrants in children should precede deep palpation. As in the adult, the area with the suspected problem should be

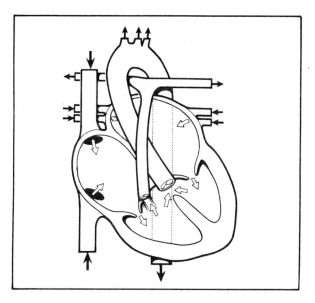

Figure 17–7C. Tetralogy of Fallot. Tetralogy of Fallot is characterized by the combination of four defects: (1) pulmonary stenosis, (2) ventricular septal defect, (3) overriding aorta, and (4) hypertrophy of right ventricle. It is the most common defect causing cyanosis in patients surviving beyond 2 years of age. The severity of symptoms depends on the degree of pulmonary stenosis, the size of the ventricular septal defect, and the degree to which the aorta overrides the septal defect.

palpated last. The child's verbal expression, crying, and facial grimaces often are used as indicators of areas of tenderness. The spleen and liver are easy to palpate in children.

Pain in the right lower quadrant (RLQ) is a frequent sign of acute appendicitis but not always specific to the diagnosis. Place the child in a supine position and have the child raise his

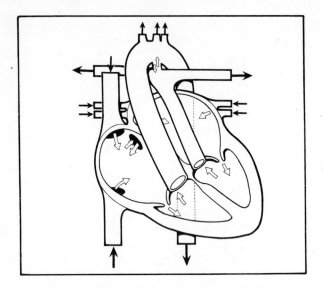

Figure 17–7D. Complete transposition of great vessels. This anomaly is an embryologic defect caused by a straight division of the bulbar trunk without normal spiraling. As a result, the aorta originates from the right ventricle and the pulmonary artery from the left ventricle. An abnormal communication between the two circulations must be present to sustain life.

or her head while the examiner's hand pushes down on the forehead, or extend the right leg at the hip as the child lies on the left side. These procedures will localize pain in the RLQ. (Figure 17–9A–D show positions for palpating the abdomen of children in different age groups.)

Adolescence

The abdomen of the adolescent is examined as in the adult.

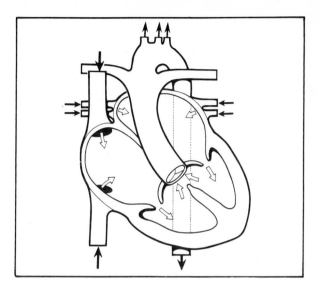

Figure 17–7E. Truncus arteriosus. Truncus arteriosus is a retention of the embryologic bulbar trunk. It results from the failure of normal septation and division of this trunk into an aorta and pulmonary artery. This single arterial trunk overrides the ventricles and receives blood from them through a ventricular septal defect. The entire pulmonary and systemic circulation is supplied from this common arterial trunk.

MUSCULOSKELETAL

Infancy and the School-Aged Child

The skeleton of the infant and young child consists mostly of cartilaginous tissue accounting for the soft, malleable bones. It is for this reason that many bone defects, identified early, can be corrected with greater ease than later in life. At birth only

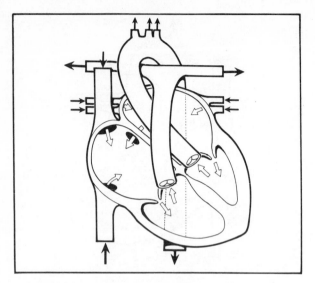

Figure 17–7F. Atrial septal defects. An atrial septal defect is an abnormal opening between the right and left atria. Basically, three types of abnormalities result from incorrect development of the atrial septum. An incompetent foramen ovale is the most common defect. The high ostium secundum defect results from abnormal development of the septum secundum. Improper development of the septum primum produces a basal opening known as an ostium primum defect, frequently involving the atrioventricular valves. In general, left to right shunting of blood occurs in all atrial septal defects.

one concave (C-shaped) spinal curve, the primary curve, is present. The secondary or compensatory curves, which give the spine its characteristic S shape, develop later. The cervical curve appears at 3 to 4 months when the infant begins to hold

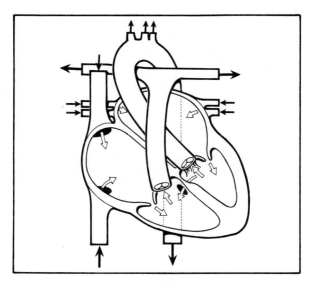

Figure 17–7G. Subaortic stenosis. In many instances, the stenosis is valvular with thickening and fusion of the cusps. Subaortic stenosis is caused by a fibrous ring below the aortic valve in the outflow tract of the left ventricle. At times, both valvular and subaortic stenosis exist in combination. The obstruction presents an increased work load for the normal output of the left ventricular blood and results in left ventricular enlargement.

up his head. The lumbar curve appears when walking is achieved at 12 to 18 months of age.

If the infant's feet retain their uterine position, they may appear to be deformed. Positional deformities can be distinguished by the ease with which the affected foot can be manipulated to neutral and over-corrrected positions. Also, stroking along the outer edge of the affected foot will cause it

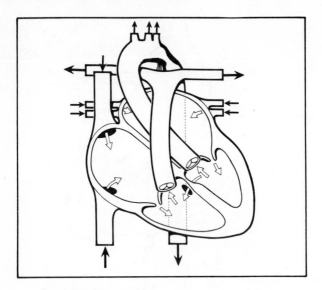

Figure 17–7H. Coarctation of the aorta. Coarctation of the aorta is characterized by a narrowed aortic lumen. It exists as a preductal or postductal obstruction, depending on the position of the obstruction in relation to the ductus arteriosus. Coarctations exist with great variation in anatomical features. The lesion produces an obstruction to the flow of blood through the aorta, causing an increased left ventricular pressure and work load.

to assume a normal position. Adduction of the infant's forefoot distal to the metatarsal-tarsal line (metatarsus adductus deformity) is a common finding and spontaneously corrects itself by the age of 2 years.

A problematic foot deformity more common in male infants is clubfoot or talipes equinovarus. This deformity may

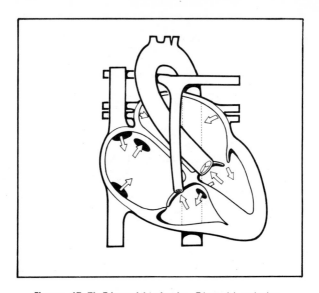

Figure 17–71. Tricuspid atresia. Tricuspid valvular atresia is characterized by a small right ventricle, large left ventricle, and usually a diminished pulmonary circulation. Blood from the right atrium passes through an atrial septal defect into the left atrium, mixes with oxygenated blood returning from the lungs, flows into the left ventricle, and is propelled into the systemic circulation. The lungs may receive blood through one of three routes: (1) a small ventricular septal defect, (2) patent ductus arteriosus, and (3) bronchial vessels.

include a severe degree of plantar flexion, heel inversion, and forefoot adduction giving the foot a backward appearance. Orthopedic referral for x-rays, plaster casting, exercises, and/or operative procedures is essential.

When the infant begins to walk, he or she may be misdiagnosed as flatfooted because the feet are set widely apart

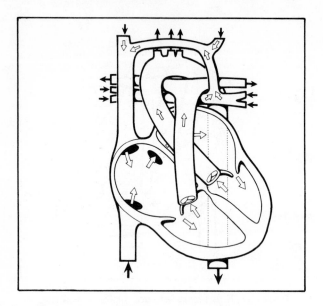

Figure 17–7J. Anomalous venous return. Oxygenated blood returning from the lungs is carried abnormally to the right side of the heart by one or more pulmonary veins emptying directly, or indirectly through venous channels, into the right atrium. Partial anomalous return of the pulmonary veins to the right atrium functions the same as an atrial septal defect. In complete anomalous return of the pulmonary veins, an interatrial communication is necessary for survival.

with weight-bearing on the inside of the foot. There is also some pronation of the foot and incurving of the Achilles tendons. With the longitudinal arch of the infant's foot obscured by adipose tissue, the foot has a flat appearance.

From early infancy to 18 months of age, a distinct bow-legged growth pattern is present. A gradual transition from bow-legs to knock-knees occurs and persists until the child is

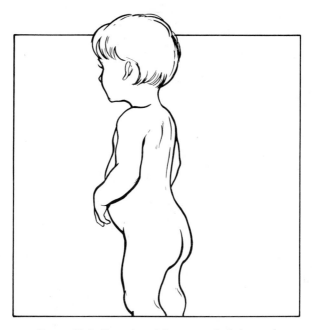

Figure 17–8. Normal protuberance of abdomen in early childhood.

about 12 years old, when a balancing takes place and the legs straighten. Twisting or torsion of the tibia inwardly or outwardly is a common occurrence that usually corrects itself by the time the child is 2 years old.

The skin folds of the thighs, gluteal folds, and popliteal creases are inspected for asymmetry (Figure 17–10), which is a sign of congenital dislocation of the hip. The extremities are inspected and palpated for symmetry, mobility, masses, and ROM. The ROM of all joints is great in infancy, with gradual

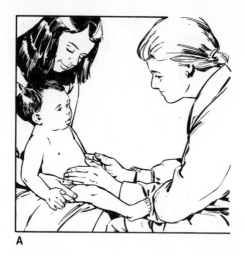

A

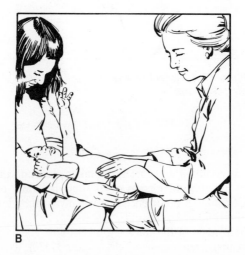

B

Figure 17–9. Positions for palpating the abdomen of children in different age groups. **A.** Palpating the abdomen of an infant. **B.** Palpating the abdomen of a 2-year-old.

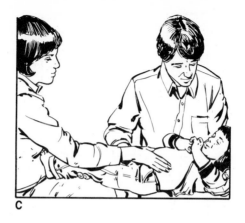

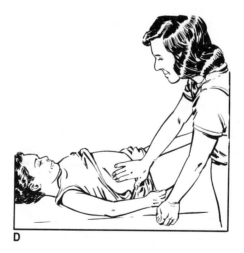

Figure 17–9 (continued). C. Palpating the abdomen of a 3-year-old. **D.** Palpating the abdomen of a 4-year-old.

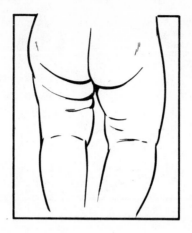

Figure 17–10. Asymmetric gluteal folds in congenital dislocation of the hip.

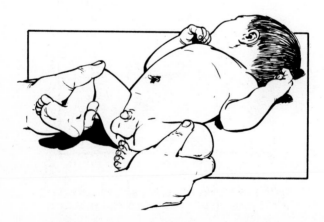

Figure 17–11. Ortolani's sign, maneuver used for detecting congenital dislocation of the hips.

diminution during childhood until the adult status is reached. Inspect the infant's hips for signs of congenital dislocation where the femur head is displaced and out of the acetabular socket. Place the infant in the supine position with the legs toward the examiner. Flex the legs at right angles at the hips and knees with passive manipulation, and abduct them until the lateral aspect of each knee touches the examining table. If congenital dislocation is present, abduction of the affected hip is limited. The examiner then performs the *Ortolani test* (Figure 17–11), by placing the infant's legs in neutral position and examining one hip at a time, using the other hip to stabilize the pelvis. Abduction, traction, and inward pressure are applied over the freater trochanter with the index and middle fingers. If a reducible location exists, a "click" in the hip will be felt. The examiner then performs *Barlow's test* (Figure 17–12) by abducting the infant's hip, using the length of the fingers to apply pressure along the axis of the femur, and producing outward pressure with the thumb. This manipulation slips the reduced hip posteriorly over the acetabulum's edge. Suspicion or identification of a dislocated hip requires orthopedic referral.

Inspect the child in several positions, standing straight with feet together, stooping, standing, and touching toes. Inspection from behind while the child shifts his or her weight from leg to leg is necessary to observe for hip disease. The pelvis will tilt toward a diseased hip when weight-bearing occurs on the affected side, but will remain level with weight-bearing on the unaffected side.

Inspect and palpate for joint pain, which may indicate trauma or tumors. Inspect for scoliosis by having the child bend forward and observing for symmetrical position of the hips and shoulders and by inspecting the spinous processes for abnormal curvature.

Adolescence
By the time adolescent years are reached, the various child-hood characteristics of the skeletal system have been replaced by the more mature, adult stature. The knock-knees and the

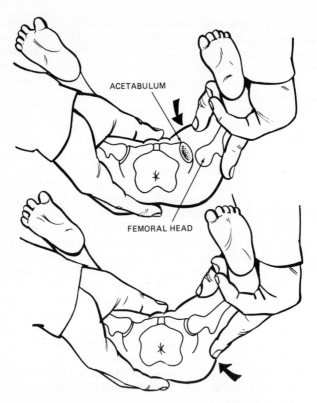

ACETABULUM

FEMORAL HEAD

Figure 17–12. Barlow's sign, maneuver used to detect unstable (nondislocated but potentially dislocated) hips.

postural slumps are gone. The feet, however, begin to show the effects of wearing different, modern styles of shoes, and corns and callouses are common findings.

Careful inspection and palpation of extremities are performed for symmetry, nodules, pain, and ROM. Because scoliosis is common in this age group, the shoulders and hips

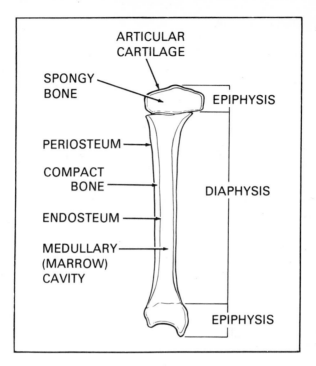

Figure 17–13. Slipped femoral epiphysis.

are inspected carefully for alteration in symmetry. True scoliosis versus postural scoliosis is assessed in the same manner as for the adult. If scoliosis is suspected, orthopedic referral is made.

If the teenager has a limp and gives no history of injury or trauma, slipped femoral epiphysis may be suspected (Figure 17–13). Any teenager with severe, persistent pain or swelling in long bones should be referred for evaluation as osteosarcoma (Ewing's tumor) occurs in this age group.

FEMALE GENITALIA

Adolescence

Examination of the adolescent female follows the same procedure as for the adult. It should be stressed, however, that both a menstrual history and sexual history are extremely important to discern any areas that may be problematic.

Precocious sexual maturation or delayed maturation in the adolescent often indicates abnormal function of the hypothalamus, pituitary, adrenals, or gonads. Precocious puberty is usually seen as the appearance of secondary sex characteristics in a young girl before the age of 8. Puberty is considered delayed if secondary sex characteristics are not apparent before age 13 in girls.

If the adolescent is sexually active, a discussion of family planning is appropriate.

MALE GENITALIA

Infancy and Childhood

The foreskin of the infant is inspected. The foreskin adheres to the glans penis and has a small orifice at its distal end. It does not retract over the glans until the infant is several months old. Most infants today are circumcised so that the glans is exposed to its base. Hypospadias is present when the urethral orifice is at some point along the ventral surface of the glans or the shaft of the penis. The testes are normally found in the scrotum. If they are found in the inguinal ring they may be easily milked down into the scrotum. If testicles cannot be palpated in the scrotum have the child sit in a cross-legged squatting position with the examiner palpating the inguinal canal and scrotum. A diagnosis of undescended testicles should not be made until the inguinal canal and scrotum are palpated with the child in this position. If the testes are palpable, no problem exists. (See Figure 17–14.)

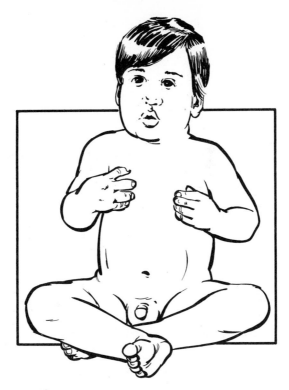

Figure 17–14. Position for palpating retracted testicles.

Precocious puberty is the appearance of secondary sex characteristics in a young boy before the age of 9 and requires referral for further investigation and treatment.

Adolescence

The genitalia in the male adolescent is examined as in the adult. It is, however, essential to evaluate the presence of the testicles in the scrotum. Undescended testicles (cryptorchid-

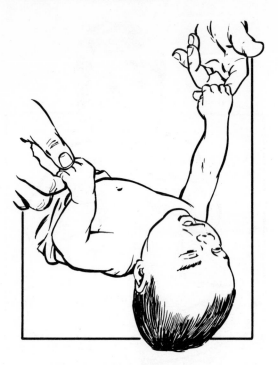

Figure 17–15. The grasp reflex.

ism) at this age may result in sterility. Secondary sex characteristics include pubic and axillary hair, increased size of testicles, deepening of the voice, penile enlargement accompanied by increase in height and muscle mass and should be evident in most boys by the age of 14. Delayed puberty beyond this age requires referral for evaluation. Sexual maturity progresses at different rates and the complete change from prepubescence to adulthood takes anywhere from 2 to 5 years.

If the adolescent is sexually active, a discussion of family planning is appropriate.

NEUROLOGICAL

Infancy and Childhood

The neurological examination of the infant requires skilled observation and inspection. It should never be performed when the infant is hungry or sleeping soundly. The quality of nervous system functioning is revealed by observing symmetry of spontaneous movements, appearance, positioning, posture, spontaneous alertness, movement of all four extremities, vigor of feeding, and responsiveness of the infant to parents and environment.

Because the child goes through an intense period of development that is related, in part, to the increasing myelinization and maturation of the neural system, the child's overall developmental progress needs careful evaluation. Measures for testing how well the neurological system is functioning include the quality, pitch, loudness, and duration of the cry; any drowsiness or irritability; and social adaptive, language, and motor skills.

The automatic infant reflexes that are normal at birth and disappear around 4 months of age are the *Moro reflex*, the *palmer grasp reflex*, and the *rooting reflex*. When these reflexes are absent, a severe problem of the CNS may exist; when they persist there may be an equally serious problem. (See Figures 17–15 and 17–16 for illustrations of reflexes.)

To elicit the Moro reflex, the examiner places the infant in the supine position and surprises him with a loud noise. The infant responds with a grasping movement; the arms extend and then flex, and the knees and hips flex. The palmer grasp reflex is obtained when the examiner touches one of his or her fingers to the palmer surface of the infant's fingers. The infant automatically grasps the finger tightly. The rooting reflex is elicited by gently stroking the infant's cheek and lips with a finger. The infant will turn the head and search for the finger.

Other reflexes are observed in infants. The tonic neck reflex (Figure 17–17) appears when the infant is 1 month old and disappears in 3–5 months. It is elicited by placing the

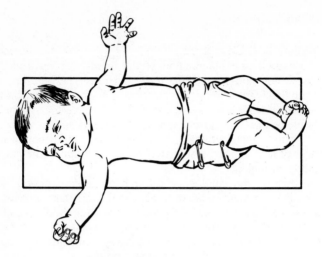

Figure 17–16. Moro reflex.

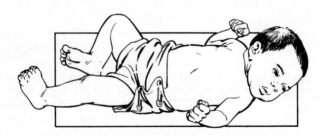

Figure 17–17. Tonic neck reflex.

infant in the supine position and turning the head to the left or right. The infant assumes a "fencing" position when the arm on the side toward which the head is turned extends and the other arm flexes.

The Babinski reflex is normally present in all infants. This reflex is demonstrated by stroking the lateral plantar surface of the foot. The infant responds with an upward fanning of the toes, which is a positive response. There is no significance to this response, but it should disappear when the infant is 9 months old. After this time, it is an abnormal finding.

Throughout infancy, specific gross motor and fine coordination testing can be accomplished by using the Denver Developmental Screening Test. This test also assesses social and language development. A discrepancy in motor and communication achievement needs further investigation to determine if it is in the motor, sensory, or intellectual spheres.

Motor function testing in the infant is achieved by putting each major joint through ROM and assessing whether normal muscle tone, spasticity, or flaccidity is present.

The sensory examination in infants is of limited use in defining neurologic disease because thresholds of touch, pain, and temperature are higher than in older children and reactions to these stimuli are low. Specific sensory function can be tested by gently touching the infant's arms and legs with a pin and observing movement in the touched extremity or change in the child's expression. It is not necessary to prick the skin and produce crying in the infant.

After 2 years of age the neurological examination of children is performed following the same methods used with the adult. Only the conversation, direction, and developmental tasks are altered to be more suitable to the child's level of understanding.

Adolescence

The examination of the adolescent's neurological system follows the same procedure as for the adult.

18 | Assessment of the Geriatric Patient

Being old may be more a frame of mind than any particular chronological age. For purposes of research some people have designated the "young-old" as 65 to 74 and the "old-old" as 75 and older. Whatever the designation of elderly, we know that life expectancy has increased and more people over 65 years are being seen in health-care settings. Thus, it is imperative that the elderly patient be recognized as having some unique characteristics that occur from anatomical and physiological changes associated with the process of aging.

Because aging does not occur at the same rate in each person, there will be great variations in physical findings from patient to patient of the same age. However, there are some well-recognized body changes that the examiner should keep in mind when examining the elderly. The more common changes that may be present in the elderly patient will be presented for each portion of the health assessment.

HEALTH HISTORY

While the principles of the interviewing process remain essentially the same for the elderly patient, there are a few guidelines to keep in mind.

1. Privacy is especially important to most elderly patients;

they should be questioned in a private examining room or in a hospital room with the curtain pulled.

2. Mental processes may be slowed, so questions should be simple, straightforward, and in lay language.

3. The interview and examination should not be rushed.

4. If a hearing loss is present, the questions should be spoken slowly and directly to the patient. (Hearing loss makes privacy in a hospital setting very difficult.)

5. For some elderly patients it will be necessary to supplement the health history information by talking to a relative or close friend. Past medical records of the patient are also useful in supplementing information of past history.

Chief Complaint

Remains one sentence in the patient's own words.

History of Present Illness

The format for the HPI remains essentially the same as for the adult patient. When the pattern of illness points to a particular health problem but the symptom of pain seems particularly lacking, recall that pain perception is often reduced in the elderly person and may obscure the diagnosis. In addition, long-standing diabetes mellitus may produce neuropathies that blunt pain perception to the point where even an acute myocardial infarction may go unrecognized.

Past History

This portion of the health history may be lengthy and complicated, depending on the number of past health problems of the patient. Areas that need recording and attention are long-standing medical problems, particularly those under current treatment (diabetes, hypertension, heart disease, cancer, and renal or liver dysfunction).

Past uncomplicated surgical procedures are of less consequence, as are childhood illnesses and uncomplicated fractures. The infectious diseases of prime importance are rheumatic fever and frequent sore throats (assuming them to be strep infections).

A thorough listing of all medicines, both prescription and over-the-counter drugs, should be made. Elderly patients often take medications long past their prescribed use or stop taking them when they feel better. Patterns of use may suggest possible toxicity or abuse, which can be explored further in the ROS questioning.

Family History
In general, the questioning can be brief, as a genetic and familial health history is of little value in the 70- or 80-year-old patient.

Review of Systems
All body systems should be reviewed, but questions that are obviously of no consequence should be eliminated. For example, a detailed menstrual and pregnancy history in a 70-year-old female is unnecessary. The number and outcome of pregnancies should be recorded along with age of menopause, but unless complications are mentioned this can be done briefly.

Patient Profile
This portion of the health history may well be the most important of all. How the elderly person cares for himself, what the usual sleep and elimination patterns are, what social support systems are available to the patient, and how the patient views himself and his life are vitally important in planning care and treatment for this age group. This portion of the health history should be done completely, following cues that provide insight into any financial or environmental factors that may affect the patient's ability to assume care for himself.

PHYSICAL EXAMINATION

Skin and Integument

Skin loses its elasticity and subcutaneous fat as it ages, thus contributing to the wrinkled, drier look of the elderly. Chronic exposure to sunlight and weather appears to hasten this process.

Three common non-malignant skin lesions found in the elderly are: *seborrheic keratoses*, *senile lentigines*, and *senile* or *actinic keratoses*. Seborrheic keratoses are raised, dark colored, warty-looking lesions with a scaly, greasy surface. These are usually located on the trunk, face, neck, and hands. Senile lentigines, also known as liver spots or aging spots, are brown flat macules, like large freckles, that appear on the backs of hands, forearm, neck, and, occasionally, the face. These spots do not fade even when not exposed to sunlight. Senile keratoses begin as small reddened areas and then become raised, rough, brownish lesions. These lesions develop on exposed skin surfaces.

Other non-pathological skin changes in the elderly are *cherry anginomes*, which are small, round red spots of clustered capillaries, and *senile purpura* or vivid purple macules or patches caused by blood leaking from capillary walls into the dermis of the skin. Neither of these findings is significant.

There is an increased chance of developing cancer in the elderly, and two common types of skin cancer are found in this population. The first is *squamous cell carcinoma* which occasionally develops from senile keratosis; the second is *basal cell carcinoma*, which appears as a papule with a pearly border and a depressed or ulcerated center.

The elderly also experience changes in their hair and nails. Hair on the scalp loses its pigment but, with the popularity of hair rinses and coloring, this may not be immediately evident. Hair texture on the scalp for both sexes will become finer and hair will decrease in number and diameter. Many men will lose their hair, beginning with thinning at the temples and progressing to the top of the head. This is a genetically determined characteristic. Hair distribution over most of the body, including the legs, trunk, axillae, and pubic area, becomes more sparse, but hairs in the nose, ears, and eyebrows become coarse and bristlelike. Following menopause some women may have coarse hairs that appear on the chin and upper lip. Because of the normal loss of body hair with age, the absence of hair on the legs, as a symptom of arterial insufficiency, may go unrecognized.

Nailbeds may thicken and yellow with age. However, very thick toenails that defy cutting are usually the result of a fungal infection or peripheral vascular disease, and not just aging. Thick toenails cause great difficulty with adequate care of the feet and proper footwear.

Head and Neck

Facial features change with age owing to wrinkling and skin laxity, the use of glasses, the graying of the hair, and dentures. All of these changes can be more or less pronounced, depending on weight gain or loss, skin exposure, and, of course, the use of makeup. Many elderly people are edentulous; if teeth are still present they may be yellowed or translucent. When dentures or partial plates are worn they should be removed and the mouth carefully examined for lesions or sores. Poor-fitting dentures are often a cause of poor nutrition and poor eating habits in this age group. When teeth are present the mouth and gums should be examined carefully for receding gum lines, inflammation, and even pockets of purulent drainage around the teeth. Periodontal disease is a major cause of tooth loss in adults. If the patient's own teeth appear worn down, it may be due to constant contact with dentures that wear away the real teeth enamel.

With the increased incidence of carotid occlusion in this population, palpation and auscultation of the carotid arteries for bruits should always be done in the examination of the neck. All cranial nerves should be assessed, recognizing that diminished hearing, sight, and smell are normal in the elderly.

Eyes

Numerous changes in the eye occur with aging. On inspection the eyelids may appear more wrinkled and hang in loose folds. This is caused by the loss of subcutaneous fat and is sometimes coupled with weakened eyelid muscles, causing a senile ptosis. With lack of skin tone of the eyelid the lids may turn in (entropion) or out (ectropion). *Arcus senilis,* or corneal arcus, is an opaque ring or arch around the edge of the cornea and is a common finding in the elderly. Some claim it is due to lipid deposits, but it is not considered pathological and does not affect vision. There is some loss of lacrimal secretion with aging and the patient may complain of dry eyes.

On opthalmoscopic examination the lens may appear cloudy or even opaque, indicating the presence of *cataracts.* Cataracts are lens that have thickened and changed in texture with age so that the passage of light is impaired. They are relatively common in the 65-year-old age group and occur with increasing incidence with advancing age. As the lens continues to enlarge over the years it may cause a narrowing of the angle between the iris and the cornea and thus increase the risk of *narrow-angle glaucoma.* Checking for increased intraocular pressure is a standard practice when patients are fitted for eyeglasses.

When the fundus is examined it will generally show narrowed and pale arterioles. In the presence of chronic diseases the fundus will show degenerative changes associated with that particular disease. Because hypertension and diabetes are so common in the elderly, the eyegrounds should be examined carefully for the presence and extent of A-V nicking and the presence and extent of diabetic retinopathy.

With all the possible changes in the visual apparatus of the eye, it is not surprising that visual acuity is usually diminished in the elderly. The most common visual change with aging is the loss of elasticity of the lens, resulting in an inability to focus on near objects (farsightedness). Such changes are usually noticed long before the 60s and the use of glasses is usually the outcome. Visual acuity, especially near vision, should be checked by having the patient read newsprint at 6 to 12 inches. Adequate vision through the use of corrective lenses, cataract surgery, or other means can greatly increase the independence and self-sufficiency of the elderly patient.

Ears

The tympanic membrane of older people may appear duller, paler, and retracted; however, the most common changes in the ear will be in loss of hearing. In most cases, hearing loss in the elderly is the result of either *presbycusis* or *otosclerosis*. Presbycusis is a bilateral loss of sensorineural function, or hearing sensitivity, usually affecting the high-frequency range (above 1000 Hz) most. The patient with presbycusis may have difficulty hearing consonants. Otosclerosis is a loss of movement of the stapes due to bony fixation at the oval window of the ear. This results in a conduction defect that is usually greatest for low frequencies. The patient with this condition may have difficulty hearing vowel sounds. Otosclerosis may be surgically treatable or helped with the use of a hearing aid.

While all patients with a hearing loss should be referred for an audiometric examination, the use of the Weber and Rinne screening tests may be useful in distinguishing conduction from sensorineural defect.

Since hearing sensitivity from 500 to 2000 Hz has been shown to be important for understanding the spoken word, the use of tuning forks at the 512 Hz, 1024 Hz, and 2048 Hz frequencies is recommended to avoid overestimating the hearing sensitivity of elderly patients. If only one tuning fork is to be used it should be the 512 Hz, as this range can more readily detect hearing loss in the lower frequencies.

Breast and Axilla

The techniques and procedures of the breast examination do not differ from that of the adult patient. The elderly female breast does change in texture due to the atrophy of breast glandular tissue. This is often described as "stringy and fibrous" on palpation. If the patient has gained weight over the years, the amount of fat tissue may have increased in the breasts, but due to the loss of connective tissue the breasts tend to sag or appear pendulous.

Careful palpation of the breasts remains of primary importance in the physical examination, as the incidence of breast cancer in the female increases with age. Patient education on the techniques and reasons for routine breast self-examination should be done. The elderly female patient will not have mensus as a reminder to plan self-examination, so another routine time, such as the first of each month, should be designated so this activity is not neglected.

Because the risk of breast cancer increases with age, mammograms are recommended for women over the age of 50.

Thorax and Lungs

The aging process results in a stiffening of ligaments, a decrease in size and resiliency of intervertebral discs, and skeletal changes that accentuate the dorsal curve of the thoracic spine. These changes often result in dorsal kyphosis with an increased A-P diameter of the thorax. While the bony changes in themselves may not impair respiratory function, functional changes that accompany aging cause a decline in vital capacity and diminish optimal respiratory capacity. The net result is less respiratory reserve even in lungs free of disease. The lungs tend to retain some mucus and the possibility of infections is increased.

The elderly are also more likely to have degenerative disc disease and arthritis of the spine, which will further contribute to inadequate lung expansion. Common respiratory pathology of the elderly includes chronic obstructive pulmonary disease and carcinoma of the lung. Patients with a history of prolonged smoking or exposure to dust or fumes in a work setting are at high risk for both of these diseases.

Normal physical findings in the elderly will include the tendency toward an increased A-P diameter and loss of vital capacity. Hyperresonance on percussion and diminished or distant breath sounds will be noted.

Long-standing habits are difficult to change, but moderate regular exercise, clean air, and no smoking can improve lung function and should be encouraged.

Cardiovascular

Cardiovascular disease is a very common health problem of the elderly. As the body ages the blood vessels lose their elasticity, become more rigid, lengthen, and form more tortuous pathways. These changes are normal and the rate and severity will vary with the individual. As these changes occur and become coupled with some degree of atherosclerosis, the lumina of the vessels decreases, and both systolic and diastolic blood pressure increase.

The myocardium may also show signs of atrophy in the aging process, with a decrease in both size and strength of the contractible force. These changes can ultimately lead to a decrease in cardiac output. In addition, heart valves become thicker and less flexible because of fibrosis. Such changes cause ineffective valve closure and produce murmurs.

Elderly people also have an increased incidence of benign premature contractions. Treatment of both of these physical signs, murmur and premature beats, should be approached constructively as they may represent only normal aging instead of treatable pathology.

While these are normal changes of aging, they can collectively place an added burden on the heart; in addition, many patients will have past histories of stress or damage to the cardiovascular system. In such patients the examiner will be particularly concerned with a careful description of all drugs the patient is taking, as patients are often on "heart pills" for long periods without supervision. Particular attention should also be paid to symptoms that may indicate a deterioration in cardiovascular status. Such symptoms include increased problems with breathing (especially associated with physical exertion), fatigue, edema of the extremities, dizziness, confusion, and syncope.

Cardiac conditions found more frequently in the elderly population include atrial fibrillation, congestive heart failure, hypertension, and dysrhythmias requiring pacemakers.

The aging process also affects the aorta and large major arteries, making them stiffer and less distensible (elastic). These changes coupled with a long-standing history of hypertension make elderly people more at risk for aneurysms and strokes. The abdominal aorta and the carotid arteries should be carefully auscultated and palpated for bruits and palpable enlargements.

Peripheral Vascular

Problems with peripheral circulation are common in the elderly. This is not surprising, considering the number who have diabetes mellitus, hypertension, and other types of cardiovascular disease. Careful attention should be paid to the possibility of both arterial and venous insufficiency, with thorough history questions and complete physical examination of feet and lower extremities.

Abdomen

The abdominal examination of the elderly does not vary significantly from that of the adult. The only point that needs emphasizing is that both neoplasms and aneurysms are more frequent in the elderly, making careful palpation and identification of masses of increased importance. Aneurysms are characterized as a pulsating mass, and bruits should be audible on auscultation. Because of flattening of the diaphragm with age, often compounded by respiratory disease, the liver edge may be more easily palpated in the elderly than in younger adults. Such a finding does not always mean hepatomegaly. To adequately evaluate if liver enlargement does exist, the span of the liver should be determined by percussion.

There are a variety of gastrointestinal symptoms that plague the elderly including constipation, anorexia, and "heartburn." A slowing in motility of the gastrointestinal tract and decreased production of gastric secretions may contribute to these symptoms. However, no symptoms should be automatically attributed to "old age" without an adequate exploration.

Musculoskeletal

Loss of muscle strength and muscle bulk due to muscle atrophy accompanies aging and is often compounded by a lack of physical activity and regular exercise in this age group. Recovery from injury is delayed because the ability to regenerate new cells is slowed.

Ligaments and joints are stiffened with the aging process, and intervertebral discs lose their resiliency. Because of these changes and the dominance of the flexor muscles, the dorsal spine becomes pronounced, resulting in kyphosis and a decreased range of motion (ROM) at the neck, back, and extremities. Osteoarthritis of the spine and weight-bearing joints of the hip, knees, and ankles is a frequent finding in the elderly, contributing to joint pain and reduced ROM.

In evaluating ROM in the elderly the examiner must be cognizant of painful joints and not contribute to the pain by too vigorous testing and manipulation of joints and extremities.

Many elderly people develop a swaying motion when they stand in one place. This swaying appears to be without a pathological basis and should be considered normal and taken into account when doing the Romberg test.

Neurological

The neurological system is primarily affected in aging by a "slowing down" of function or a decrease in acuity rather than any marked change in neurological status. Although cognitive abilities can be diminished, this is usually a result of disease processes such as arteriosclerosis, organic brain syndrome, Alzheimer's disease, and the like. Contrary to popular belief, severe mental illness occurs in less than 10 percent of the population over 65 years of age. However, varying degrees of mental impairment result in considerable concern and cost for many families of the elderly.

In addition to the changes already mentioned in hearing, vision, and smell, common neurological changes associated with aging include diminished deep-tendon reflexes, diminished or lost abdominal reflexes, loss of vibratory sense in ankles and feet, and, less commonly, a loss of proprioception, contributing to an unsteady and often wide-based gait. It is important to keep in mind that while such changes are often the result of the normal aging process, changes that are asymmetrical are abnormal and deserve further investigation.

Problems with gait can occur for a variety of reasons; for the most part, abnormal gaits represent disease conditions, and for the elderly these are usually Parkinson's disease, arthritis, cerebellar disease, or post-stroke paralysis.

Loss of balance is not a normal sequel of aging; thus, a careful attempt should be made to establish the cause of this problem.

Male Genitalia

As already noted, pubic hair decreases in elderly males and may become gray; the penis may also decrease in size. These are normal changes and do not necessarily correlate with a decreased libido. The elderly have a higher incidence of benign prostatic hypertrophy, carcinoma of the prostate, and carcinoma of the rectum, and for this reason a digital rectal examination should always be included in the physical examination for the elderly male, and the stool checked for occult blood.

Female Genitalia

Following menopause (approximately 40 to 55 years of age) and the subsequent decrease in estogren production, there are several changes that normally occur in the female genitalia. The external structures including the labia and clitoris become smaller and the introitus is reduced. The internal organs (uterus, cervix, and ovaries) all decrease in size, making the ovaries rarely palpable on bimanual examination. The vaginal mucosa thins, secretions are reduced, and the vaginal vault is shortened and less elastic. This drier, thin-walled vagina may result in erosions, ulcerations, and painful intercourse (dyspareunia). Vaginal creams may help this condition, but the routine administration of estrogen to prevent these atrophic changes in post-menopausal women is discouraged. Estrogen and progesterone supplements may be used, depending on the individual patient's needs and health history. Whenever such therapy is initiated, careful follow-up is required to monitor possible side effects, including the development of neoplasm.

Finally, because the most feared disease of the reproductive system in the elderly is carcinoma, Pap smears and routine pelvic examinations are encouraged on a yearly basis. Some women believe (falsely) that after menopause such examinations are not necessary, and this is not the case.

19 | Selected Laboratory Findings

TABLE 19-1. COMPLETE BLOOD COUNT

Test	Normal Values	Selected Abnormalities
Red Blood Cells (RBC)	Male 4.5–6.0 million/mm^3	↑Polycythemia vera
	Female 4.0–5.5 million/mm^3	↑Severe dehydration ↓Hemodilution after blood loss ↓Anemia (see RBC indices)
Hemoglobin (Hgb)	Male 14–18 g/100 ml Female 12–16 g/100 ml	↑Severe dehydration, hemoconcentration ↓Anemia, leukemia
Hematocrit (Hct)	Male 40–54% Female 37–47% Generally Hct = 3 × Hgb ± 3%	Same as above
Reticulocyte Count	0.5–1.5% 25,000–75,000 cell/ml	↑Bone marrow hyperproliferative, ie, hemolytic anemia, lymphocytic leukemia, systemic lupus

(continued)

TABLE 19-1. COMPLETE BLOOD COUNT (Continued)

Test	Normal Values	Selected Abnormalities
		↓Bone marrow hypoproliferative, ie, iron deficiency, pernicious anemia, folic acid deficiency
Erythrocyte Indices Indirect Mean Corpuscular Volume (MCV)	82–92 μm^3	↑Macrocytic anemia, ie, folic acid deficiency, pernicious anemia ↑Normocytic anemia, ie, chronic renal failure, cancer, acute or chronic infections, chronic liver disease ↓Microcytic anemia, ie, iron deficiency anemia
Mean Corpuscular Hemoglobin Weight of $\dfrac{Hgb}{RBC}$ RBC	27–31%	↑Macrocytic anemia (rarely used) ↓Microcytic anemia
Mean Corpuscular Hemoglobin MCHC $\dfrac{Hgb}{Hct}$ %	32–36%	Normal value = normochromic Low value = hypochromic
White Blood Count (WBC)	5,000–10,000/ml	↑Acute infections ↓Agranulocytosis (see differential for more specific information)

TABLE 19-2. W & B DIFFERENTIAL

Differential	Relative Value	Absolute Value (WBC × Rel. Val.)	Selected Abnormalities
Neutrophils (in order of development stages)			↑Infection, granulocytic leukemia
Myeloblasts	0	0	↓Mumps, measles, hepatitis, anticonvulsants, antihistamines, sulfonamides, some antibiotics, aplastic anemia, agranulocytosis
Premyelocytes	0	0	
Myelocytes	0	0	
Metamyelocytes	0	0	
Band (non-segmented neutrophils)	0–10%	0–1,000	
Segmented neutrophils	60–70%	3,000–7,000/mm^3	
Monocytes	2–6%	100–600/mm^3	↑T.B., bacterial endocarditis, monocytic leukemia
Lymphocytes	20–40%	1,000–4,000/mm^3	↑(Many viral infections) mumps, German measles, infectious mononucleosis, viral hepatitis, lymphocytic leukemia ↓Stress from trauma, burns, epinephrine, ACTH, cortisone
Eosinophils	1–4%	50–400/mm^3	↑Allergies, asthma, skin diseases ↓High levels of insulin, epinephrine, ACTH
Basophils	0.5–1%	25–100/mm^3	↑Granulocytic leukemia, irradiation, hemolytic anemias, splenectomy

TABLE 19-3. ELECTROLYTES

Tests	Normal Values	Selected Abnormalities
Sodium	136–142 mEq/L	↑Decrease water intake ↑Excessive oral or I.V. intake of sodium ↑Diabetes insipidus ↑Sodium bicarbonate given in cardiac arrest ↓GI suctioning ↓Vomiting ↓Diarrhea ↓Adrenal insufficiency ↓Excessive infusion of nonelectrolytes
Potassium	3.5–5 mEq/L	↑Renal failure ↑Following severe burn ↑Blood sample left sitting too long ↑Adrenal insufficiency ↓Metabolic and respiratory alkalosis ↓G.I. Loss—diarrhea, vomiting, NG suctioning ↓Potassium wasting drug therapy
CO_2 combining power	24–30 mEq/L	See bicarbonate under blood gases
Chloride	95–103 mEq/L	↑Acute renal failure ↑Renal tubular acidosis ↓Congestive heart failure ↓Diarrhea ↓Adrenal cortical insufficiency

TABLE 19-4. BLOOD CHEMISTRY

Tests	Normal Values	Selected Abnormalities
Amylase	60–160 (Somogyi units)/100 ml	↑Pancreatic disease
Alkaline phosphatase	30–85 IU	↑Post-hepatic obstruction ↑Viral hepatitis ↑Infectious mononucleosis ↑Metastatic bone cancer
Acid phosphatase	0–1.5 U	↑Acute and chronic renal disease ↑Accompanies high alkaline phosphatase in metastatic prostatic carcinoma
BUN (Blood urea nitrogen)	8–18 mg/dl	↑Renal failure ↑Dehydration ↑GI hemorrhage ↑Congestive heart failure ↓Cirrhosis of liver
Calcium	9.0–11.0 mg/dl (4.5–5.5 mEq/L)	↑Primary hyperpara-thyroidism ↑Cancer of lung, kidneys ↑Hyperproteinemia ↑Acidosis ↓Low albumin levels ↓Hypoparathyroidism ↓Alkalosis
Creatinine	0.6–1.2 mg/dl	↑Congestive heart failure ↑Chronic glomerulo-nephritis
Cholesterol	150–250 mg/dl	↑Cardiovascular disease ↑Hypothyroidism ↑Nephrosis ↑Uncontrolled diabetes ↑Obstructive jaundice ↓Portal cirrhosis

(continued)

TABLE 19-4. BLOOD CHEMISTRY (Continued)

Tests	Normal Values	Selected Abnormalities
Lipoprotein		
LDL	73–200 mg/dl	↑Atherosclerosis CAD (coronary artery disease)
HDL	32–75 mg/dl	↑Exercise Low-fat, low-cholesterol diets Alcohol intake
Triglycerides	10–190 mg/dl	↑Uncontrolled diabetes ↑Obstructive jaundice ↓Portal cirrhosis
Total Bilirubin	0.2–1.2 mg/dl	↑Hemolytic jaundice ↑Hepatic jaundice ↑Post-hepatic obstructive jaundice
Conjugated (direct) bilirubin	0.1–0.2 mg/ 100 ml	↑Marked in post-hepatic obstructive jaundice ↑Normal in hemolytic jaundice
Unconjugated (indirect) bilirubin	0.1–0.6 mg/ 100 ml	↑In hemolytic jaundice
Uric acid	Male 2.1–7.8 mg/dl Female 2.0–6.4 mg/dl	↑Gout ↑Infectious mononucleosis ↑Chemotherapy for cancer ↑Renal failure
Proteins (total)	6.0–7.8 g/dl	↑Lupus erythematosus ↑Acute liver disease
Albumin	3.2–4.5 g/dl	↓Inadequate protein intake ↓Nephrosis ↓Burns ↓Portal cirrhosis
Globulin	2.3–3.5 g/dl	↑Portal cirrhosis ↑Multiple myeloma

TABLE 19-5. ENZYMES

Tests	Normal Values	Selected Abnormalities
CPK (creatine phosphokinase)	Male 20–90 IU/L Female 14–60 IU/L	↑Within 4 hr post-myocardial infarction ↑Muscular dystrophy ↑Muscle trauma
LDH (lactic dehydrogenase)	80–120 (Weeker units) 150–450 (Wroblewski units)	↑Within a day and peaks in 4 days' post-myocardial infarction
SGOT (serum glutamic oxyaloacetic transaminase)	8.33 U/ml	↑Acute liver disease ↑Acute renal disease ↑Acute myocardial infarction
Glucose	70–110 mg/dl	↑Diabetes mellitus ↑Brain trauma ↓Excess insulin administered to diabetic ↓Psychogenic conditions
Phosphorus	3–4.5 mg/100 ml	↑Chronic nephritis ↓Renal tubular acidosis

TABLE 19-6. URINALYSIS

Test	Normal Values	Selected Abnormalities
Bacteria count		If shows ↑ bacteria with no WBCs, redo test
Color	Yellow, clear	
pH	4.6–8.0	
Specific gravity	1.016–1.022 (normal fluid) 1.001–1.035 (range)	If shows ↑ bacterial with WBCs, do a culture and sensitivity
Glucose	0 neg	
Albumin	0 neg	
Blood, occult	0 neg	
WBCs	0	
Bacteria	0	Usually treat if bacteria > 100,000 and WBCs present
Total volume/ 24 hr	600–1600 cc	
Urine urobilinogen	0–4 ml/24 hr	↑Hemolytic jaundice (normal value in post-hepatic obstructive jaundice)
Urine bilirubin	None	↑Post-hepatic obstructive jaundice (none in hemolytic jaundice)

TABLE 19-7. BLOOD GASES

Arterial Blood Gases	Normal Values
pH	7.35–7.45
pO_2	80–100 mm Hg
O_2 saturation	95–100%
pCO_2	35–45 mm Hg
HCO_3^-	22–26 mEq/L (is also reflected in CO_2 content in electrolyte results)

Blood Gas Abnormalities

7.35–7.45 pH	35–45 mm Hg pCO_2	22–26 mEq HCO_3^-	Assessment
↓	↑	normal	Respiratory Acidosis
↑	↓	normal	Respiratory Alkalosis
↓	normal	↓	Metabolic Acidosis
↑	normal	↑	Metabolic Alkalosis
↓	↑	↓	Mixed Resp. & Metabolic Acidosis
↑	↓	↑	Mixed Resp. & Metabolic Alkalosis
↓normal	↑	↑	Compensated Respiratory Acidosis
↑normal	↓	↓	Compensated Respiratory Alkalosis
↓normal	↓	↓	Compensated Metabolic Acidosis
↑normal	↑	↑	Compensated Metabolic Alkalosis

TABLE 19-8. COAGULATION TIME

Coagulation Tests (see also Figure 19-1)	Normal values
Bleeding time (Ivy)	1–5 min
(Duke)	1–3 min
Clotting time (Lee-White)	7–15 min
Prothrombin time (to be compared with control)	12–14 sec
Activated partial thromboplastin time (PTT)	35–40 sec

Anticoagulation Drugs

Heparin		**Coumadin**
Anticoagulant drug interferes with thrombin formation		Interferes with liver absorption, synthesis, and storage of vitamin K
Peak 20–30 min Duration 4 hr		Depresses factors II, VII, IX, X
Anticoagulant therapy levels 2–2½ times normal blood values		Onset 10 hr Peak 2–5 days Duration 10–14 days
Continuous IV 60–100 sec q 6 hr	PTT 55–75 sec	Anticoagulant therapeutic levels 1½–2½ times control of Protime about 20–30 sec
Coagulation time (Lee-White)	30–45 min	

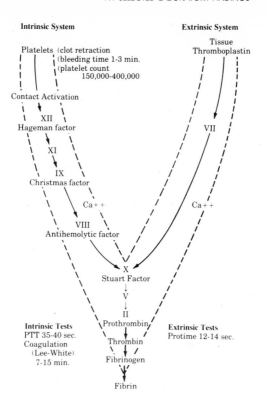

Figure 19–1. Coagulation pathway.

The ECG

TABLE 20-1. ECG CONFIGURATIONS

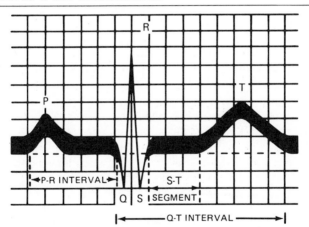

Electrical pattern of cardiac cycle

p wave	< 0.10 sec
	Best seen in Lead II
	Represents atrial depolarization
PR interval	0.12–0.20 sec
	Shows conduction through AV node, bundle of His, bundle branches
QRS complex	0.06–0.10
	Represents ventricular depolarization

ST segment	Normally at isoelectric line
QT interval	0.36–0.44 sec
	Represents ventricular systole, depolarization, and repolarization of ventricles
T wave	Upright curve except in AVR
	Represents ventricular repolarization

Isoenzymes for Myocardial Infarction

An isoenzyme is a varied molecular form of a particular enzyme. Each isoenzyme is specific for one particular organ tissue. Therefore, with tissue damage, enzymes are spilled into the blood system and with electrophoretic separation the organ responsible for the enzyme elevation can be identified.

In acute myocardial infarctions, the isoenzymes of lactic dehydrogenase (LDH) and creatine phosphokinase (CPK) are most frequently used to determine the presence of an infarction.

Creatine Phosphokinase (CPK)
or Creatine Kinase (CK)

There are three CPK isoenzymes, with CPK-MB present in the myocardium. Following an acute myocardial infarction (MI) CPK-MB, or CPK_2, is elevated 4 to 8 hours after chest pain, and reaches peak activity at 18–24 hours. The presence of CPK-MB with a greater quantity than 5% of total CPK or greater than 10 IU indicates myocardial damage. CPK_2 is also found in the serum of patients with other cardiac disorders and certain neuromuscular disorders.

Lactate Dehydrogenase (LDH)

Lactate dehydrogenase can be divided into five isoenzymes. Cardiac muscle is rich in LDH_1, an isoenzyme that is also present in the kidney and red blood cells. Normally the isoenzyme LDH_2 is present in the blood serum in greater

TABLE 20-2. ECG ABNORMALITIES IN MYOCARDIAL INFARCTION

ECG Pattern	Figure
Normal ECG pattern (A)	
Ischemia—Depressed or inverted T wave (B)	

A

B

(continued)

TABLE 20-2. ECG ABNORMALITIES IN MYOCARDIAL INFARCTION (Continued)

ECG Pattern	Figure
Injury—ST segment elevation or depression (C)	
Necrosis—Q wave (D) To be considered pathological Q waves must be: New Finding Duration 0.04 sec or longer Usually 4 mm or greater in height Appear in leads that do not usually have Q waves	

C   D

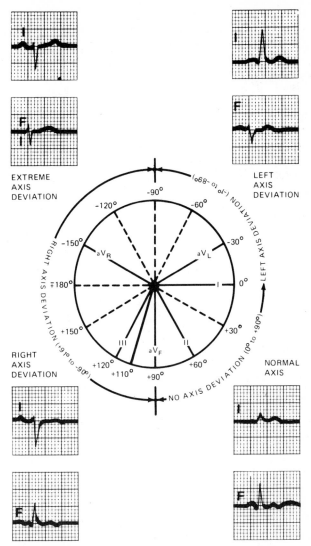

Figure 20–1. Axis deviation.

concentrations than LDH_1. However, with myocardial tissue damage the ratio becomes reversed, or "flipped," and LDH_1 is in higher concentration than LDH_2.

In the presence of myocardial damage, the LDH assumes the flipped profile usually 21 to 24 hours after the acute episode. This flipped pattern is also seen in acute renal infarction, and in hemolysis associated with prosthetic heart valves, hemolytic anemia, and pernicious anemia. However, the LDH flipped pattern with the proper clinical picture is usually diagnostic of an acute myocardial infarction.

Summary
In a patient with the proper clinical picture, the presence of CPK_2 in the serum followed by the LDH flipped pattern is nearly 100% predictive of an acute myocardial infarction.

Axis Deviation
The orientation of the heart's electrical activity in the frontal plane is termed "axis." The axis can be determined from any two limb leads. Using limb leads I and aVF and looking at the positive (+) or negative (−) deflection of the QRS complex, you can place the axis in its appropriate quadrant. See Figure 20–1 for quick reference.

A more precise location of axis can be achieved by comparing the size of the QRS complexes in the two leads, plotting them on the axis chart, and drawing a horizontal line through the aVF point and a vertical line through the Lead I point. Where the two lines intersect will be the electrical axis.

BIBLIOGRAPHY

Andreoli K, Zipes D, Wallace A, et al.: *Comprehensive Cardiac Care* (6th ed.). St. Louis: CV Mosby, 1987.

Bates B, Hoeckelman RA: *Guide to Physical Examination and History Taking* (4th ed.). Philadelphia: J.B. Lippincott, 1987.

Cancer Facts and Figures. New York: American Cancer Society, 1989.

Carroll-Johnson RM (Ed.): *Classification of Nursing Diagnoses: Proceedings of the Eighth Conference (NANDA)*. Philadelphia: J.B. Lippincott Co. 1989.

DeAngelis C: *Pediatric Primary Care*. (3rd ed.). Boston: Little, Brown, 1984.

DeGowin RL: *DeGowin's and DeGowin's Bedside Diagnostic Examination* (5th ed.). New York: Macmillan, 1987.

Delp MH, Manning RT: *Major's Physical Diagnosis: An Introduction to the Clinical Process* (9th ed.). Philadelphia: W.B. Saunders, 1981.

DeVita V, Hellman S, Rosenberg S: *Principles and Practice of Oncology* (3rd ed.). Philadelphia: J.B. Lippincott, 1989.

Eliopoulas C: *Health Assessment of the Older Adult*. Boston: Addison-Wesley, 1984.

Fox JA: *Primary Health Care of the Young*. New York: McGraw-Hill, 1981.

Fitzpatrick J, Kerr M, Sabo V, et al.: Nursing Diagnosis: Translating Nursing Diagnosis into ICD Code. *American Journal of Nursing* 89:493, 1989.

Groenwald SL: *Cancer Nursing*. Boston: Jones and Bartlett, 1987.

Guzzetta CE, Bunton SD, Prinkey LA, et al.: *Clinical Assessment Tools for Use with Nursing Diagnosis*. St. Louis: CV Mosby, 1989.

Halsted CH, Halsted JA: *The Laboratory in Clinical Medicine: Interpretation and Adaptation* (2nd ed.). Philadelphia: W.B. Saunders, 1981.

Harvey AM, Johns RJ, McKusick V, et al.: *The Principles and Practice of Medicine* (22nd ed.). Norwalk, CT: Appleton & Lange, 1988.

Henry JB (Ed.): *Todd-Sanford-Davidsohn: Clinical Diagnosis by Laboratory Methods* (17th ed.). Philadelphia: W.B. Saunders, 1984.

Hurley M (Ed.): *Classification of Nursing Diagnoses: Proceedings of the Sixth Conference* (NANDA). St. Louis: C.V. Mosby, 1986.

McClintic JR: *Physiology of the Human Body* (3rd ed.). New York: John Wiley, 1989.

Malasanos L, Barkoukas V, Stoltenberg-Allen K: *Health Assessment* (4th ed.). St. Louis: C.V. Mosby, 1989.

Rudy E: *Advanced Neurological and Neurosurgical Nursing*. St. Louis: C.V. Mosby, 1984.

Sherman J, Fields S: *Guide to Patient Evaluation: History Taking, Physical Examination & the Nursing Process* (5th ed.). New York: Elsevier, 1987.

Smith LH, Wyngaarden JB: *Cecil Review of General Internal Medicine* (4th ed.). Philadelphia: W.B. Saunders, 1989.

Taxonomy I. Revised (1990) with Official Diagnostic Categories: St. Louis, North American Nursing Diagnosis Association.

Tilkian AG, Conover MG: *Understanding Heart Sounds and Murmurs* (2nd ed.). Philadelphia: W.B. Saunders, 1984.

Tilkian AG, Conover MG, Tilkian AG: *Clinical Implications of Laboratory Tests* (4th ed.). St. Louis: C.V. Mosby, 1987.

Whaley LF, Wong DL: *Nursing Care of Infants and Children* (3rd ed.). St. Louis: C.V. Mosby, 1987.

Widmann FK: *Clinical Interpretation of Laboratory Tests* (9th ed.). Philadelphia: F.A. Davis, 1983.

INDEX